Secrets Behind Energy Fields

Become Your Own Energy Guru
Reclaim Energy and Vitality

MYRA SRI

www.myrasri.com
Energy Healing Secrets Series

Copyright and Legal Notice

This Book is Copyright © 2015 and Beyond: Myra Sri (the "Author"). All rights reserved worldwide.

Reproduction or translation of any part of this work beyond that permitted by section 107 or 108 of the 1976 United States Copyright Act without permission of the copyright owner is unlawful. Requests for permission or further information should be addressed to the Author. No part of this Book may be translated or reproduced or transmitted in any form or by any means, electronic or mechanical, including photocopying, recording, or by an information storage and retrieval system without the express permission of the Author.

This publication is designed to provide accurate and Authoritative information in regard to the subject matter covered, based on the Author's experience, research, practice and understandings. The Author and publisher do not recommend anything contrary to common sense. If professional medical or nutritional advice or other expert assistance is required, the services of a competent professional person should be sought.

First Published as electronic book in Australia 2012
First Printing Revised: **August 2015**
Published by Healing Knowhow™ Publishing,
P.O. Box 126, Toukley, NSW 2263, Australia

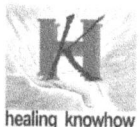

National Library of Australia Cataloguing-in-Publication entry
Sri, Myra, author
Secrets behind energy fields : become your own energy guru, reclaim energy and vitality / Myra Sri
ISBN; 978-0992392420 (paperback)
Energy healing secrets series ; 2
Energy medicine
Includes bibliographical references
615.89

Acknowledgements

Thank you to my clients, students and colleagues for your encouragement with this endeavour.

Amazon Reviews

"Thanks to this eBook, I am teaching myself to rise above the conflict at work... these life skills are priceless!"

"This is an excellent, practical, down to earth book that is filled with simple techniques to get in touch with yourself, your own energy, what is affecting it and then how to do something about it."

"I found this book very informative and the techniques were simple and easy to follow. I would recommend it to anyone who does energy work."

Book Includes:

What to do when others drain you

How to rebuild your aura and energy fields

The 3 most common energy problems

How to handle energy difficulties

Easy how-to Self-Test instructions

How to clear other's 'dumps' from energy fields

And much more...

Other Books by the Same Author:

Energy Healing Secrets Series

Secrets Beyond Aromatherapy

Secrets Behind Energy Fields

Secret Truths to Health and Well-Being

Secrets to Serene Space – Space Clearing

New Crystal Codes

Guided Meditations at www.myrasri.com/new-healing-store

OTHER AMAZON BOOK REVIEWS:

"A treasure of energetic information"

"Thrilled with the content of this book and I have read almost every aromatherapy book there is"

"I wonder why this book is not used as a textbook."

Contents

INTRODUCTION 11
ABOUT THIIS BOOK 15

PART 1 BEHIND THE ENERGETICS OF THE HUMAN ENERGY SYSTEMS 17

EVERYTHING YOU NEED TO KNOW 19
   TO INCREASE YOUR HEALTH POTENTIAL, AND MAINTAIN RESILIENT ENERGY BOUNDARIES 19
   FIRST THINGS FIRST: 20
   THE HIDDEN TRUTHS BEHIND EXHAUSTION REVEALED! 23
      Relief After Extended Stress 23
      Hidden Feelings 25
      Pain Avoidance 28
      Denial Can Kill You 29
      Inner Conflict 30
   RESULTS OF POOR PERSONAL BOUNDARIES 32
   PERSONAL BOUNDARIES 35
      1. Our Personal Belief Systems 35
      2. Family Dynamics 35
      3. Others 36
      4. Partner 36
      5. Peers 36
      6. Self – Abuse 37
      7. Self – Un-Awareness 37
      8. Self – None-Belief 38
      9. Self – Doubt 38
   IS ALL THIS REALLY NECESSARY? 40

ENERGY FIELDS AND SYSTEMS 43
ABOUT YOUR PERSONAL ENERGY SYSTEMS 47
   PHYSICAL BODY SYSTEM 49
   EMOTIONAL BODY 51
   MENTAL BODY 54
   ASTRAL BODY 56
   PSYCHIC BODY 57
   MORE ON ENERGY, HUMAN ENERGY FIELDS & AURA 60

THE SCIENCE OF THE AURA 63
   THE AURA AND ELECTROMAGNETICS 63
   A WORD ON ELECTROMAGNETICS 64
   PERSONAL FREQUENCIES 50
   BIRTHPLACE ENERGY BOOSTERS... 72
   GALACTIC FREQUENCIES 73
   SEEK PEACE... 73

PART 2 SELF HELP YOURSELF - EXERCISES YOU CAN START NOW!...75
   STRENGTHENING YOUR ENERGY FIELDS — CREATE RESILIENCE 77
      COMMON REASONS FOR WEAKENED ENERGY FIELDS........... 78
      STRESSFUL SITUATIONS OR EVENTS 78
HOW TO MANAGE YOUR OWN ENERGY AND SPACE TO BE AROUND OTHERS WITHOUT FEELING DRAINED 81

ENERGY ENHANCING EXERCISES.. 83
   SOLAR LIGHT - PROTECTION 83
   RECALL AND REALIGNMENT OF PERSONAL ENERGY.............. 85
   RECALL OF PERSONAL ENERGY EXERCISE 87
   RECALL OF SELVES 88
   DEALING WITH TOXIC PHONE CALLS... 89
     1. Green Ear Muffs:.. 89
     2. Green Column 91
     A Third option 92

3 PROVEN WAYS TO STRENGTHEN YOUR AURA, INCREASE ENERGY AND CREATE RESILIENCE..93
     1. THE PSYCHIC BODY TONER... 94
     2. RECOGNISE THE POWER OF ESSENTIAL OILS TO STRENGTHEN YOUR ENERGY SYSTEMS................................... 97
     3. HOW TO USE ESSENTIAL OILS TO STRENGTHEN YOUR ENERGY SYSTEMS... 99
   Oil Meditation Technique 100
   Oils to Strengthen Energy Systems and Create Resilience . 102

ENERGY SEPARATION ISSUES... 107
   THREE MOST COMMON ENERGY PROBLEMS 107

PREPARE FOR RESTFUL SLEEP - **111**
    5 PROVEN STEPS TO SEPARATING YOURSELF FROM UNSETTLING ENERGIES.. 111
    WORKAHOLICS OR WORRIERS, A CLOSING DOWN PROCESS IN CASES OF INSOMNIA 113
    PORTAL & REALITY CLOSING DOWN PROCESS 114
    SLEEP SUGGESTION.. 116
    AN EASY WAY TO CLEAN UP TOXIC ENERGIES.................... 117
    TOXICITY CLEARING EXERCISE: 100
    GOLDEN GATES 1188

SECRET TECHNIQUES AS QUICK PICK-ME-UPS **125**
    NECK CLEANING AND NECK SCARF...................................... 126
    MAGENTA COLUMN AND WHITE CIRCLE.............................. 127
    TO FURTHER SUPPORT ENERGETIC PROTECTION 129
    SHOPPING CENTRE PROTECTION:... 130
    A WORD ON PERSONAL PROTECTION —THERAPISTS........... 130
    QUICK START RECIPE FOR GOOD BASIC ENERGY SYSTEM SUPPORT 132

PART 3 HOW TO KNOW YOURSELF — AND KNOW OTHERS... **135**
    THE FINGER TEST SELF HELP TECHNIQUE........................... 137
        How To Clean Up After Others Have Dumped On You 137
        The Steps.. 138
    THE FINGER TEST SELF HELP TECHNIQUE........................... 140
        The Secret 142
    CLICK" AND "FLICK" FINGER TESTS 144
        IMPORTANT! 147
        Train the Brain... 149

HOW TO IDENTIFY USING THE FINGER TEST **151**
    HOW TO IDENTIFY WHAT IS BOTHERING YOU THAT YOU HAVE PICKED UP FROM BEING AROUND OR FROM HEARING OF OTHERS PROBLEMS OR ISSUES (AND HOW TO DEAL WITH THEM) 151
    ASK THE RIGHT QUESTIONS: 153
    TAKE THE RIGHT ACTION - STAY ENERGETICALLY SEPARATE: 155
    STRATEGIES TO CLEARLY IDENTIFY YOUR ENERGY PROBLEM 156
    SECRET WAY TO IDENTIFY WHAT IS BOTHERING YOU.......... 161

How To Clean up After Others Have Dumped On You
— and Maintain Your Energy 162
    The Steps 162
Disposal of Toxic or Unwanted Energies.................... 163
Disposal Of Negative Thoughtforms........................... 165
Your Secret Weapon 166
Practicing Being Aware... 167

PUTTING IT TOGETHER.. 169
A Guide — Ideas / Invocations 171
Some Contaminations To Test For — "Is This True?" . 171
A List Of Statements To Test 173
Further Statement Ideas to Test 174
Create Your Own Favorite Statements: 176
A Guide - List Of Common Statements 177
Where To Next?... 179
    The Challenge 180
    Next Step 182

Further Information 185
    Questions & Contact Information 186
    Resources... 186
    Disclaimer..185
About the Author 189

Secrets Behind Energy Fields

INTRODUCTION

Many of us lead busy lives. Many of us are involved with others whether at work, on the social front or with family. Many of these interactions with others can inspire, energise and rejuvenate us. Some can relax and refresh us.

And some can exhaust us. Or worse.

When we don't know where our energy goes, when we work with others closely, when we are faced with emotional or traumatic scenes, when others think it is ok and acceptable to explode around us, when we think there must be something wrong with us because of what we continually encounter in our life, to survive without going nuts we need answers to what is happening and what we can do about it!

Over the years I have experienced energy drain, exhaustion to the point of severe depression, mind-fug and headaches due to other minds trying to get into my head, emotionally toxic people and despair at the inhumanity man doles out to his or her fellow 'man'.

Things got so bad because I hadn't realized my energy systems had been compromised. At one stage I was so overwhelmed almost to the point of an identity crisis partly because of what I was picking up from others pains, hurts, angers, fears and frustrations and partly because I was giving too much of myself and didn't know how to protect my own energies and stop letting others demand from me or take from me.

Now that is the hard and pointy end of the stick. Not everyone experiences energetic drain and interference to the same degree. There are varying degrees of sensitivity, and I was pretty sensitive. And I had to do some major learning about all of this and how to not only prevent it, but also repair the damage done.

Having said that, however, doesn't mean that other people haven't experienced what I have. They just may not have recognised it, and simply thought they were tired for "doing too much", or felt that there was a fault within themselves for "not coping".

Nobody lives as an entire isolated and energetic island to themselves. We are all social beings and part of life is social interaction of some kind or another.

Learning to navigate through life in energies that are less than positive sometimes requires outside information or help.

Many others have come to me with similar problems and because of my own experiences and searchings I have had answers for them - and I hope to share with you some of these practical and proven techniques, easy exercises, effective solutions and self empowering tools for the weary, the overwhelmed, the sensitive, the long-suffering and the compromised.

These techniques are suitable for all those who experience the following:

> If you want to know how to save a whole lot of money using natural methods to feel better and in a drug-free-way

> If you feel that they are overtired and overwhelmed by life's duties and responsibilities but don't know how to stop the merry-go-round

> If you feel others take advantage of you and you don't know how to avoid this

> If you don't know what to do around toxic people

> If you are looking for answers and aren't happy with what you've been told by others so far

...Then just maybe this book holds some answers for you.

Secrets Behind Energy Fields

As an energy worker, facilitator and instructor for over 25 years, I have had to learn the hard way how to support my own personal energies and health whilst being around others who were themselves in trouble. The information and techniques in this book are distilled from many years of training, practice and life experience.

When we have good health, we really do have a huge asset at the ready – there is no price to be placed on it as from our good health so many positive things can arise. And all you really need to invest is some of your time and energy to become your own guru and healer.

To be successful and happy, let good health and good energy be your positive foundation.

Secrets Behind Energy Fields

ABOUT THIS BOOK

This book is in three (3) parts or sections, with a Summary section

Part 1

- Know and Respect Your Personal Energy
- All about your Personal Energy Fields and Energy Systems and Their Impact on Your Health and Energy

Part 2 –

- Strengthening Exercises You Can Start NOW that will Make-All-The-Difference
- All about the Reasons for Weakened Energy Systems, Energy Exercises and Secrets

Part 3

- How to Clean Up
- How to Self-test - Your Amazing Self Help Tool
- Real Energy Secrets – Your Own Personal System that will give you Your Answers!

Summary – Putting It All Together

- Statement Lists

REMEMBER THIS:

Energy is more than just eating right...

There is an ENERGETIC component that is often ignored.

For Energy to be available, "on tap" as it were, the energy lines MUST be clear. There should be no overload or we may overwhelm or "blow a fuse". There must be protection along the lines so that the energy does not "leak" away. There should be access to the Energy source for the supply to continue.

So here is my response to questions, real problems by real people and requests to "get it out there to help others". You are welcome to contact the writer with other specific problems that have not been included. There is a complete workshop that includes the ideas in this book and more called "HygienEthics", specifically designed for those who are sensitive or have been traumatized in some way.

It's time to take a look at the Energy Dynamics or Energetics of Energy, exhaustion and hidden energy problems...So let's get started.

PART 1 BEHIND THE ENERGETICS OF THE HUMAN ENERGY SYSTEMS

- Personal Boundaries and impacting issues
- Know and Respect Your Personal Energy
- All about your Personal Energy Fields and Energy Systems and Their Impact on Your Health and Energy
- The Aura
- Impact of Emotion
- Reasons for Exhaustion, Fatigue and Tiredness

Myra Sri

Everything You Need To Know

To Increase Your Health Potential, and Maintain Resilient Energy Boundaries

This book is all about your Health and your Personal Energy. In these pages you will discover how to know and respect your energy fields, and how to create strength and resilience.

You will find exercises to strengthen your health and energy, and tips and tools to assist your energy fields to be strong enough to be fully functioning and self sustaining again.

The state of your energy systems directly reflects upon your health. Maybe not immediately, which is why we can function under tremendous pressures for a time. But the cost will come because you will be losing energy, and will not be recharging it again. There are many reasons for energy drains and depletions, and in this book we cover the common and most frequent issues.

At differing times in life, we don't have the same energy we had previously, and we may find it really hard to feel okay when interacting with others.

Experiencing a trauma will change the "tone" or health of our energy fields. Whilst dramatic change thrust upon us and even continual stress will also affect our energy fields in detrimentally - unless we take steps to clear, recharge, heal or balance them back to health again.

We may have experienced a shock, a serious illness, a series of unsettling experiences, a loss, a huge or forced change in circumstances, or we may have been thrust into something similar by supporting a very dear or partner, family member or close friend. Over time, we eventually recover, but it may take quite a while to do so, and if the circumstances surrounding us are not favorable to supporting this recovery, we may feel that we are going round in circles.

There is a growing need for people to be able to not only recover their sense of being okay around others, to improve their ability to understand or identify the things that affect them, but to give them the power to be able to take responsibility for keeping their energy systems strong, and to be able to protect themselves from being drained by others or by difficult situations or circumstances.

The bottom line is that you don't really need to know anything about your energy fields for these techniques to work.

You can even skip this part, and you can still use all of the information in this book accurately and effectively.

But if you really want to know more about how you function energetically, and you are willing to benefit from the knowledge of those who have seen, felt, and worked directly with energy fields, and who have documented and refined their findings, then you can profit from this effort and work. Discover your Energy Fields, how they impact on your health, what affects them and how. And what you can do about it.

FIRST THINGS FIRST:

Firstly, some information on the components of the Energy Systems or Energy Fields, as these govern your available energy supply. Then we will look at what we can do to protect, strengthen, support and them clean up.

We refer to both energy fields and systems together in this book, as the energy systems support the energy fields

Secrets Behind Energy Fields

and also because one is dependent on the other; like a generator supports the lighting and electrical appliances in a household or business, so the systems continually affect and supply the tone or wattage of energy fields. Our main concern here is how to maintain clear energy charges for correct functioning of a healthy energy field.

The most common reasons for loss of energy and weakened Energy Systems will be exposed, and you will begin to learn to discover for yourself just what affects you personally. This can be very valuable information for many reasons.

Take a moment to imagine this:

Remember feeling flat and drained in the past when you were with certain people?

...

Now, just imagine that they no longer have any effect on you!

...

How does that feel? Just think about it...

...

How would it be if they never affected you like that again?

...

That is what I want you to take away with you in this book.

So take notice of what you read, and PUT IT INTO PRACTISE!

The tools and knowledge you need are ALL provided.

The Hidden Truths Behind Exhaustion Revealed!

Fatigue, Exhaustion, Always Tired?

Let's look at some of the Hidden Truths behind exhaustion that are of an energetic nature. What I mean by that is that they are not necessarily or primarily of a physical cause.

Many complain about feelings of exhaustion. There are multiple reasons for this, and most of us are already aware of many of them.

A lot of us are becoming more aware of when we are doing too much. Some of us can literally work ourselves into the ground if we aren't careful. We can also "serve" (others) too much possibly to our own detriment or harm.

Another obvious reason for exhaustion is either the lack of nutrition, or the lack of proper processing of our nutrition, such as compromised digestive assimilation or faulty hydration. Toxicity that has gone unrecognized can also impact on the brain, nervous system and body. I write more fully about this in "Secret Truths - Health and Well-Being".

Besides these obvious explanations there are other more subtly hidden causes, hidden truths. I would like to share these with you.

Magnesium Deficiency

Many are not aware of the need for the important mineral magnesium. It is one of the most significant minerals in all bodily processes. One little known secret is this; It is also absolutely *essential* for sensitive type people and for those who care a lot. Engaging with others requires a *huge* amount of unseen energy, and we can literally "chunk through" our magnesium supply unless we replace it regularly.

Psychics and intuitive types, as well as counselors and "people people" also use a lot of this in their energetic interactions and in their thought processes. Ensuring that you have enough magnesium will also enhance your hydration, which supports the brain and the total nervous system!

Relief After Extended Stress

Have you ever noticed when you have been in a crisis or when someone close to you has been going through one, how you feel relieved when it is finally all over? We can have an amazing surge of energy for it feels like a weight has been lifted.

Then within a matter of hours or days, we feel like a limp rag. We wonder where those amazing relieved feelings have gone. Even when we think the positive thoughts that gave us a surge of energy, it doesn't actually stay unless we think those thoughts *continually*. In effect this seems to lessen their intensity... and the intensity of those "feel-good" feelings.

A friend won a lot of money after having had years of privation. Did this solve all of her problems? Did her energy rise back up so she felt on top of the world all the time? Did her body shake off the effects of having to do without?

The answers to this are a mix of "yes" and "no" – she felt temporarily good, it alleviated her stress and the pressures placed on her, and she was on an emotional roller coaster for a while.

But at the end of it, she was still exhausted, and it took some time for her to recover from the intensity of her win, *as well as* the intensity of the years she had had to do without.

This is not to say don't try and win something. Not at all! This is to let you know that when you get those feelings of weakness, that sense of exhaustion, there is nothing at all wrong with you, it is just the process of the body releasing all of the stress it has held within it in order to get you through the situations you found yourself in.

The body has found a safe place to relax in, and now can let go of all the things it has been holding onto that it couldn't deal with before.

Survival mode causes the body to shut down on certain tasks it has in order to "ride out" or deal with the current situation. Long distance runners don't feel the need to relieve themselves when they have set their goal to run to.

People running from warring areas can put off having to eat or going to the toilet temporarily whilst they are in danger – the body allowing its systems to be put at the ready for the immediate needs of escaping in order to stay alive.

The cost of all this can be enormous. When we find a place or space to have our immediate needs met, we can "relax" whilst our bodies seek to rebalance again, but it can only do so to the extent of what is available to help it, and of how safe we are to allow it to do so.

Hidden Feelings

Sometimes the hidden reason is found in the expression of a lethargy or a repressed anger (against life or our self) that may even have a basis in depression. We often fight against this.

In my experience and studies, I have found Depression is often genetic, inherited from either one parent, or even both. It often originates with an ancestor who has undergone extreme stress or trauma or been totally unable to express themselves.

Sometimes it is not obvious, and parents have learned to hide it, choosing to "get on with it" and doing their best to "be there" for their family, children or business. But the symptoms can be recognized through their lack of happiness or a lack of peace or joy and is often coupled (though not necessarily always) with a need or addiction for distraction, relationship-chasing, drama or reality-avoidance-substances such as alcohol or social self medication.

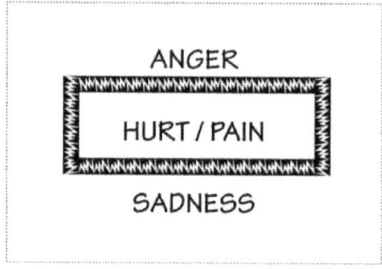

Often coupled with this and sometimes behind this is the inner struggle with hidden pain or hurt, usually from a past experience, suppressed past feelings or confusion over the unhappiness or despair that they feel from time to time.

This hurt or pain is covered or veneered with a more acceptable response of sadness or anger, like a sandwich.

The outer covering of sadness or anger protects the pain.

People will generally either express the sadness of the pain, or the anger at or caused by the pain. Generally men express anger more quickly than the sadness, for this is more acceptable than the collapse into sadness which can be hard for a man to emerge back from again. Whereas women tend to the sadness more than anger. Again, this is usually because it is a more gender acceptable emotion or expression. When women get angry they are labeled quite differently from men, who can hide behind "passion". Men find it harder to hide behind "moody" or "sensitive" than women.

So generally, when something triggers or comes close to any of the components of the buried hurt or pain, male reactions can be based on the associated anger. And women's responses can be more readily associated or expressed as sadness, based on a sensitive reaction to felt pain and the hurt that has surfaced or been triggered.

We all experience fear and pain. And we can all experience the fear of pain. We have associations with past experience that warns us of similarities, and so these can trigger us into a pre-empting of experiencing the same hurt again. And this continues until we deal with the buried emotional charge associated with past experiences, past hurts, past pains.

Understanding this about our self can assist us to understand what sometimes drives other people when their reactions seem out of proportion with the current situation or reality.

But it does not help us to deal with the sudden explosion of intense feeling and often negative energies associated with these past buried pains that have suddenly erupted like the bursting of built-up septic around a wound that has only part healed on the surface.

Learning how to take care of this energetic residual energy is important for us to manage our own energy and health, particularly when dealing with those who either don't want to sort through their issues, or who don't know how to, or who wish to project these onto others.

Pain Avoidance

As mentioned it is common and natural for people to tend to avoid pain, though often going to great lengths to do so.

It is common that either anger or sadness may well be expressed as a preference first, or even both alternately, rather than to acknowledge, seek out, process, accept and then heal the underlying pain.

Refusal or avoidance to accept that pain can easily become a part of life, and then when it appears to eventually pass, and life seems to return to "normal" again or becomes easier on the surface, we may think it is over, but in reality we may well not have actually deal with it.

In order to avoid the pain, and dealing with the pain, we can make all sorts of "reasons" or excuses, and may even go into feeling sorry for our self, or into getting angry with someone else. We may well stay like this until we deal with or resolve the original pain.

[And we can even add further layers to the pain by not dealing with this original pain.]

All of this can create inner conflict, as we reach out for something more pleasant, different, safer, yet when something approaches this sensitive area, we may well push it away for fear of feeling the pain again, and only demonstrate our safer or more accepted side of either anger or sadness.

It takes a lot of energy to ignore something that is there.

Exhaustion is caused when there is an inner conflict like this.

Secrets Behind Energy Fields

Denial Can Kill You

Let me tell you a true story. A friend had been hanging out for a holiday but could not manage to get the time off work for a few years because of the needy state of the business he worked for. He took to taking doses of panadeine, paracetamol or similar daily to offset his headaches, and refused all and any advice about this – even off his wife who was a nurse. No longer a young man, he worked himself hard, and he knew he was very stressed and tired, and needing a rest.

Eventually he managed to organize to get time off work and had a celebratory lunch on the Friday, then had the whole weekend to pack for the holiday before the Monday when he would be on his first official day's holiday. Driving his wife to work that Monday for her last half day before they went off on their planned trip away together, he suffered a series of heart attacks as he drove. Being a nurse, his wife recognized what was happening and managed to get him to hospital quickly.

He didn't survive.

The cost of him continually ignoring his headaches and of taking too much over-the-counter medication, together with finally getting the time off work to just stop and relax was too high a price to pay. It became clear after his passing that his intense commitment to his job, together with his perfectionist attitude had made his co-workers very fond of him. He had driven himself till all hours – but he paid the ultimate price.

His first real holiday was the first chance his body had had to begin to "right" itself and dealing with the fall-out and effects from stressful factors in his life was just too much to be processed.

Of course, the message that too many pain killers had also impacted on his heart should not go unnoticed here, but the point here is that where there is physical pain, then there is a reason, a warning; and headaches should never just be dulled with medication without proper medical advice.

Inner Conflict

A number one reason for exhaustion is inner conflict.

Exhaustion comes when we continually fight against our self. This conflict uses up a lot of energy and tires us. We tussle with holding back our unpleasant feelings because we either don't know how to safely express them or because we are ashamed of them, or even because they may scare us.

If we are forced to go to work and we hate our job, we will be fighting our self, being even tired-er than the job normally would make us.

The same goes for if we are in an unhappy relationship. "Blowing up" does not solve this problem. We may get to temporarily express our anxiety, fear, hurt, anger or emotions, but we don't necessarily deal with the real problem. Which could be really due to our own unhappiness or resentments.

Or we may feel that we are forced into our position and then we find our attitude does not help us to handle this well.

Deeper solutions need to be found.

Inner conflict demands, and takes, our energies as we end up fighting our self. We may want something, yet resist the change necessary to have it, or to create it.

A sure sign we are in inner conflict is if we are fighting others a lot...

This <u>will</u> weaken our energy fields. Remember;

Secrets Behind Energy Fields

The energy system or aura does not need protection or strengthening unless it has been weakened!

When it has been weakened, then we need to repair it and strengthen it.

Not only so we have to strengthen it, we have to work on healing our pain, our attitudes, our history, and of letting it go and opening to new and better experiences.

To do this, we require healthy energy fields.

To have healthy energy fields, we have to heal our pain and open to new beneficial experiences.

This may look like a never ending cycle, but let me assure you that it is not. You just have to decide to start somewhere, and wherever you start changes everything anyway. Working from either side of this conundrum in honesty and sincerity with one's self, will bring great self understanding, and this can only strengthen us.

A *decision* to make a positive change, no matter where it starts, allows change to start to happen.

Strengthen the energy field from within and you increase your natural protection.

Even just reading this can start change in your mind, your heart and your energy, and you will begin to see inner solutions even if you don't yet consciously know how to "sort it".

Awareness is already happening within you and so within your energy fields. Even just reading this chapter aloud to yourself a few times can initiate positive change in your energy fields regarding this. Don't underestimate the power of the spoken or written word.

So where and how are you in conflict?

What is it you have to change in your life, beliefs or attitudes?

RESULTS OF POOR PERSONAL BOUNDARIES

Just some of the results of the above lack of proper personal boundaries can result in:

    Buried Anger or other strong emotion

    Sustained anxiety not dealt with

    Running away from conflict or commitment

    Over-involvement in the affairs of others - meddling

    Feelings of powerlessness and lack of control in life

    Wanting to avoid being wrong

    Wanting to control in order to avoid being controlled

    Inner conflict over relating with certain people

    Over focused on being liked by everyone

    Continually (or often) being angry or upset

How we feel and what we think about our self will mirror in our energy fields.

A weak picture of who we think or feel we are will result in a weakened energy, providing little boundary or resistance from other's problems, issues, thoughts, feelings, emotions or even from another's will to invade.

Other more forceful people will find it easier to gain control of or manipulate a situation to their own benefit. It also means that we have little resistance if someone wants to deliberately further their own aims at a cost to our self.

For those in intimate relationships who feel that there partner might be impacting on them or their boundaries, you may find the exercise on The Golden Gates in the

Secrets Behind Energy Fields

Prepare for Restful Sleep section may be of assistance, or at least begin to provide you with more clarity regarding the energy dynamics between you both.

General problems that come under the heading of "Personal Boundaries" follow here numerically for easy identification.

If you don't have power in your own life, someone else will!

Ask yourself some of the following questions and see what your answers are. Then look at how you can change things.

Secrets Behind Energy Fields

PERSONAL BOUNDARIES

The following list of things that can cause weakness in our energy fields can be addressed when we firstly recognize them, then when we take action to correct them. Some questions may well be asked that we have not yet answered in a way that supports our energy systems and our health. Consider them as avenues to pursue in order for greater self (and other) understanding.

Issues that are running or compromising a healthy protection of our energy fields would include issues related to:

1. Our Personal Belief Systems

What do we believe we deserve and how are we used to being treated? What new choices are we able to make to take care of our self?

Does this belief serve me?

Do I get a pay-off from this belief?

2. Family Dynamics

How has the family always done things? What pressures or expectations are we still trying to fulfill for them? How will our "changing" from the familiar family way of doing things challenge or upset them (family)? How loyal must we be to earn or to keep their love or acceptance? How much do we need to belong? How important to us is it to belong? Have we been relegated to a family role such as "black sheep", "rescuer", "not heard"? Have family approval, etc

3. Others

Do we still take too much notice or show too much concern over what others may think, monitoring our behavior accordingly? Do we think others know better than us, or that they are better than, or even that they are less than us? Do we think that they are more important than us? Are we labeled as "bad" or difficult if we speak or stand up for our self? Do we need to impress or lie to feel accepted? What is it we do to gain attention or approval?

4. Partner

Are we overly in-dependent, too co-dependent or have we reached an inter-dependent state? Are we allowed to be our self safely with our partner? Are we both in touch with and each responsible for our own issues, whilst accepting (when asked for) the support and assistance of each other? Is the relationship healthy or are we doing the major portion of giving or "fixing" continually? Or are we taking things out on our partner simply because they are available to do so?

Do I really trust myself to make the right decisions for myself? And then for the relationship? Am I heard?

5. Peers

See Others. Peers often present intense pressure, as there is usually our need to belong or for recognition, so we may put up with offensive or abusive behavior to be accepted.

Mature individuals are able to relate to their peers, without feeling pressured by them or their standards.

Do I compromise myself for acceptance? Do I stand out to be different because I need attention? Do I need to be Special in order to be seen or visible?

6. Self – Abuse

A conscious or unconscious belief that we deserve abuse can often lead us or leave us in unhealthy situations. Often past family or life experiences and patterns have imprinted on us and we find it hard to expect something better.

Statements made in our hearing, or labels given when young may have taken hold within the subconscious, yet only have been a passing opinion or judgment. It is important to recognize this, and question that label – is it really true? Are we really bad / stupid / lazy / uncreative / clumsy etc. Or was this a projection of someone else's own denied failings? Or unthinking remarks?

Getting clear of the truth or validity of a statement for our self is to begin the process of healing or of choice and change rather than condemnation. Only then can we reclaim our identity and power of self, and of self-protection.

Do I do anything that harms my sense of well-being or my body? Do I give my decisions and power away to others?

7. Self – Un-Awareness

It may often seem easier and safer for us to blame others, family, partner etc, or even to deny that we are living in a toxic or even dangerous relationship or that we may be relating in a toxic manner, than to do anything about it.

It may also be safer for us to deny that anyone could possibly be draining or energetically abusing us in any way. (Observing our behaviors before and after encounters can lead to greater self-awareness. Self awareness practice will help us to discover the truth.)

Do I avoid confrontation by not asking for change in case there is conflict? Do I put up with things, so as not to rock the boat and upset the current system? If so, what is it I am getting out of it?

Am I honest with myself, or just choosing to defend my partner/s or my own actions so as not to change? Am I scared of change?

8. Self – None-Belief

Not believing in one's self is a common and dis-empowering belief to carry. Like Catch 22, whatever we do, we are doomed.

This often and usually occurs because our parents or a close and intimate relationship didn't believe in us, or was always putting us down. Self belief **can** be reclaimed.

Do I choose to believe in others more than myself? If so, why?

Do I think I cannot do it on my own? What will happen when I choose to believe in myself and follow through?

9. Self – Doubt

Just like not believing in one self, self-doubt causes many hesitations in decision making. And it can allow others to make our decisions for us and consequently to be seen in our eyes as being more right or powerful.

Have I been put down by others? Were they absolutely right?

By what authority or superior knowing or by whose standards were they qualified to be "right"?

Secrets Behind Energy Fields

What will happen when I choose to back myself? Can I support me, be loyal to me, just like I can support or believe in others?

Can I trust myself enough to know that it is okay to make mistakes, for that is how I learn?

Is All This Really Necessary?

Okay, So I Have An Aura. Why Do I Need To Protect Or Strengthen It? If It Was Okay 3 Days Ago, Why Is It Not Okay Now?

You have already learned about some of the Energy Bodies within the aura, so anything that benefits these will benefit the aura, and so benefit the person.

In a way, the aura is an early warning system by the registering of imbalances within the separate energy fields, before it becomes illness or disease within the physical body.

You will also have read that the aura is a living system of electrons and protons. As the body is in continual motion, even when it's just lying down (the digestion is still working, and the lungs are still breathing, and the heart is still pumping), this energy surrounding the body is also in motion, though when we are resting, it may be more settled. But we are still breathing etc, so there will always be energy movement.

Just remember the components of the energy fields… And also remember that when we are <u>thinking</u>, we are engaging the mental body. And what we think about dictates the energy movements in that energy body. And that energy body will interact with and affect the emotional body, and so on…

So you see, our aura is truly in perpetual motion. The aura does not usually need protection unless it has been weakened!

And the converse is true: **If the Aura has been weakened, it needs Protection!**

We not only have to strengthen it, we have to protect it until it is strong enough to look after itself.

Secrets Behind Energy Fields

This also means that we may need to look at our own internal thinking to see if we have created the weakness within.

It is not only others and their mean-nesses or nastiness that may cause a problem, it is also what we do to our selves, or what we let others do to us.

If you don't have power in your own life, someone else will!

Myra Sri

ENERGY FIELDS AND SYSTEMS

[Know Yourself To Help Yourself]

You may be aware of some of the information here, but I am including it anyway as a basic referral point and possible confirmation of your current understandings.

It may also help those who are still learning about the energy fields and systems and want to understand more. Those who have already learned about these aspects of energy can use this section as a reminder or primer.

Our Energy Field is dependent on our Energy Systems – they "power up" if you like the charges that support the Energy Fields – problems can occur in both the energy field and in the energy systems. One such energy system is the Meridian System. Another is the Chakra System. As this is a large subject, and to avoid confusion we will simplify the information and deal with both the energy fields and the energy systems generally as one unit, unless discussed or described separately.

The very first thing that you can do is to pay attention to your Energy Fields.

We take care of our cars, our homes, our clothing. We pay attention to the fuel we put in our bodies, or in our car engines. We are aware of what we wear, of who we want to impress or even sometimes to shock.

But we often neglect understanding who we are inside, how we work as a total system, what makes us really feel good about who we are (without it being at the expense of others), and we can sometimes avoid responsibility for treating our self with respect.

Respect is a recognizing and an honoring. Are you being respectful to yourself? Or are you allowing others to pressure you? To make you do things that in your own heart you don't really want to do or don't agree with? Are you letting others make your decisions for you? Force their opinions upon you? Do you not feel strong enough to stand up for what it is you really want, or to stand up against something you find distasteful or potentially harmful?

We are not going to make any judgments about what has happened to you in the past or present here. There really is no labeling of right or wrong in this, no making something "good" or "bad", just the recognition of what happens when you are around certain others, which is often actually just a reflection of how we view or treat ourselves. This can become a really handy "mirror" reflecting back to us how the world sees or treats us, based on how we treat our self. I mention this here, because how you treat yourself will govern a lot of the tone or strength of your energy fields, and thus its ability to rise to the challenge when you need it to.

Sometimes it is how we see or feel about our self that creates a weak energy field.

Sometimes because of something that has happened to us, this weakens our energy field and makes it hard for us to respect our self and stand up for our self.

And so the cycle continues – until we change it. And today, as you read this book, you are going to learn how to change it.

Firstly <u>wanting</u> something better for your self will start you off on a road that will bring you eventually to <u>having</u> something better for yourself.

Then becoming responsible (together with strength to be able to do so) will allow you to let others "off the hook" of you wanting or wishing they would "take care" of you, for you will be able to do so by yourself. The strength to do this can be yours by practicing what you find in this book.

Secrets Behind Energy Fields

One more word on Respect. You will be clearing away from your energy fields or systems unnecessary aspects of others, and when you come to releasing these, you don't *need* to get upset or angry about it, because it's possible that *you* yourself may have to deal with the responsibility that even your emotions or even parts of your energy fields may have been passed on to others. This is not about blame, but about strengthening who you are in the best way possible.

About Your Personal Energy Systems

The Energy Systems referred to in this book generally means or includes the whole or any part of the person's total energy systems, and their aura and can include (but is not limited to) the following:

    Physical Body System

    Emotional Body

    Mental Body

    Astral Body

    Psychic Body

The term "Energy Fields" incorporates at least one or more of the following energy bodies.

There are further subtle energy systems or sub-systems, but for our current purposes, the ones listed here are the most common that we need to work with and to be aware of. So that we have a basic understanding of these aspects to the personal energy fields and how they relate to each other, it is necessary to give some information for a uniform reference.

Secrets Behind Energy Fields

PHYSICAL BODY SYSTEM

The Physical Body is obviously the part of the Energy Fields or system of a person that we can all see, unless compromised visually. We can touch it, and study it easily.

It includes the skeletal system, musculature and ligaments, the organs and glands, nervous system, circulatory system, immune system, digestive system, hormonal system, respiratory system, lymphatic system, nervous system, urinary system, reproductive system, integumentary system (skin) and all of the cells that comprise the human body system.

It works with a variety of messengers that allow function and movement of and within the body, which includes neuro-transmitters, hormones and enzymes. However, in this book we are concerned with the Physical Body Energy Fields.

This energy field, like the body itself, is generated or supported through the normal physiological functionings of the physical body which allow utilization of nutrition, water, oxygen and the benefits of sunlight etc.

The Physical Body Energy Field, like the body, responds to touch, and is part of our protective mechanism. It also responds to pleasurable sensations and it is disturbed when the body is harmed or damaged. In some systems it has been referred to as the Etheric Body, and is like the scaffolding which holds and sustains physical life.

Also connected with the Physical Body is a separate subtle energy system that is now being recognized by new developments of precision energy measuring systems. These are now confirming the ancient science passed on by Traditional Chinese Medicine of subtle energy channels in the body called Meridians. These are like tracks of energy woven through the human body that correlate to organs, systems and emotions.

When these meridians are not working effectively or their circuits have been "blown" or short-fused, then it is simply a matter of time for problems to show up on the physical level. They are often early invisible indicators of possible physical malfunctions. The related organ or area can keep going for a while, but eventually may well succumb through dis-ease.

Secrets Behind Energy Fields

EMOTIONAL BODY

The Emotional Body is not so obvious to the naked eye. Like a series of Russian Dolls, the Emotional Energy Body sits within, through and around the Physical Body, surrounding it completely in a healthy person. It sits at differing distances from the body according to race and genetic history. If you could see it, it would look like a uniform cloud of constantly swirling color, which reflects the emotion/s currently being experienced, ranging from colors clear and bright (healthy), to hues muddy and dark (problems, pain, damage etc).

It is very easily affected by imbalances in chemical intake, such as recreational drugs or certain medications, which also have a huge impact on the other aspects of the Energy Fields. The initial "lift" does not compensate for the eventual effect.

We can often recognize physical shifts or changes in emotions from the physical body by:

>   changes in posture,
>
>   facial expression, tone and colour
>
>   voice tone,
>
>   temperature,
>
>   choices in interactive normal response and manner.

The Emotional Body is not normally seen, yet some people are empathetic enough to sense when something has shifted or changed emotionally in another, even though there may be no obvious visual clues. They may be able to sense passive or hidden anger, sadness, depression, anxiety or excitement.

All you need to really know is that emotions are simply energy in motion – **e-motion, energy in motion**.

Emotions register in the central nervous system and the brain to trigger chain reactions. Reactions in the Emotional Body affect the Physical Body.

Thoughts can also register and trigger emotions. It's like a cycle.

It's amazing how someone else's emotions can immediately trigger emotions in another who was in a totally different mood previously. You can see this in audiences, sports crowds, or when someone you are hanging out with or care about gets either very good or very bad news. One <u>VERY</u> important thing to remember is that you are *not* your emotions and that emotions *do* pass.

When someone else is angry, whether obviously so or not, if you yourself have buried away some anger or pain within, it is easy for it to get triggered again. Because this anger energy is projected out from the person it may well affect and connect with the anger you hold and hide within, and it may be a struggle not to experience or express it, too. To varying degrees, this can be said of most emotions.

If you continually lock emotions away, so as not to experience them, you can make the mistake of assuming that they have disappeared.

Some emotions can be transitional, but some can become layer upon layer of unprocessed or unacknowledged energy, a bit like allowing rubbish to accumulate rather than clearing and washing up – eventually you will create a kind of stagnation within the energy field, and will find yourself becoming numb or even filling up with uncleared or ignored emotions that you may well be unable to feel at all, which often leads to a kind of apathy. Until triggered.

Or until the supposed and hoped for "death" of these unwanted emotions causes a kind of dying within the

Secrets Behind Energy Fields

energy systems themselves or even into the physicality of the body itself, with the proven possibility of un-ease and dis-ease eventually leading to disease.

Seems a safe response, this ignoring, but it can sometimes be far from safe.

Emotions are often <u>passing</u> energy experiences when they are not denied, and finding appropriate ways to allow these energy experiences to flow through and out (if they are negative or uncomfortable) is a valuable tool to have in life.

One doesn't have to let everyone know at all times what one is going through, but one does need to be able to recognize and respond appropriately to emotions, for this will increase the enjoyment of life and extend life health.

Mental Body

The Mental Body lies around and within the previous bodies, and sits generally approximately 5" – 9" from the body. In a healthy and balanced person, it is like clear rays of yellow or golden light, radiating and extending round the whole body. It expands when one is engaged in deep or focused mental processes.

It can however, pick up or be affected by a "thoughtform" that can cling to this energy field. If these are of negative origin, when you have been around someone very sad, you may also feel sad even though you are still not in their presence. That is because the thoughtform will have at its core a collection of thoughts that are capable of triggering one's own associated experiences, perceptions and emotion/s, and you will "hear" these thoughts as your own, think that these thoughts are yours, and they will in turn activate your corresponding emotional responses.

Often, one negative thought will lead to another negative thought because of engaging with these thoughtforms, so for someone who has felt rejected they might hear inner thoughts like "I am not good enough", which can be immediately followed by "no-one cares about me"", "nobody stays around for me", "they all leave me", "here we go again" and so on.

The thoughts may not be these exactly or in this above order, as I am giving you an example only. But they will nevertheless pass through the mind so quickly that we often don't even hear them, but end up feeling really bad or upset.

Recognizing that we have picked up a thoughtform can help us to understand that just as we picked it up, we can get rid of it again, and don't have to tolerate holding on to it, or continue to engage it.

Secrets Behind Energy Fields

Have you ever noticed when you have helped someone by listening to their problems, and letting them think out loud? Often they walk off feeling much better, but you may well find yourself worrying over something yourself, or feeling how they were feeling earlier.

This transference of energy (or even a thoughtform) has affected both your Mental and Emotional bodies and over time, with sufficient unrecognized and un-prevented transference of these energies, the Physical Body will become sick.

If your Mental Body (and your other energy fields) are really healthy, you will generally be able to withstand and reject these negative thoughtforms, so they cannot affect you, and retain the positive thoughtforms that make you feel comfortable and positive.

We deal with what to do about these negative thoughtforms soon.

Astral Body

This too, is not visible to the naked eye. It sits around the above energy fields, and extends approximately 6" – 13" from the body.

When people are engaged in love relationships, this energy field arcs to surround and connect with the loved one. It is a beautiful energy field of color that becomes infused with a soft rose pink color when love or romance is engaged.

We can be interested in someone we have never met before, and when standing next to them this field is engaged, and communicates without language about compatibilities and possibilities.

This energy field will also be affected when a love relationship is over, or the object of our desires or affection does no longer return our love in kind.

The Astral Body can be compromised and even damaged through the use or overuse of most recreational drugs and certain medications.

The Astral Body is not necessarily solely connected with the Astral Level, which is recognised as being in the Fourth Dimension. This is a place often visited during sleep, day-dreaming, and when working on creating something. However, one can see the strong possibility of the connection between romance and desire regarding a loved one in relationships.

Secrets Behind Energy Fields

PSYCHIC BODY

Because of the evolution and development of the Psychic Body and because of the impact upon the state, health and energy of the being when this energy body is compromised, it is included in this section. The Psychic Body is not usually individualized amongst other models of energy fields and the components of the aura. And many are somewhat confused into thinking that Psychic Body is mostly the Third Eye. This is certainly no longer the case.

The Psychic Body is generally comprised of specific energy centers (both "in-body" and "out-of-body"), and if one area or center is not fully functioning, it can well affect the whole. Or at the very least it can affect both the quality of interpretation of information, within and without of the being, and the being's ability to translate information via the "senses".

Some of the energy centers within the Psychic Body may be confused with existing Chakras but they are *not* part of the Main Chakra System.

In many systems or models, the Main Chakra System was originally acknowledged as seven; base, sacral, solar plexus, heart, throat, third eye and crown. Some systems now number them as eight due to their recognition of the Navel Chakra which they include. The Navel Chakra exists, but belongs to another Chakra system. However, whether you work with seven or work with eight "Main" Chakras is really a personal preference. This confusion or convergence over the last twenty years or so simply demonstrates the developing awareness of other Chakras besides the original seven.

For the last thirty years, there has also been an evolution in the Human Energy Systems, and particularly within the Psychic Body.

This exponential leap is so huge and clear that it is currently being documented for inclusion in my new book: "The New Evolved Chakras". With the advent of the new millennium and in particular the click-over year of 2012, our energy systems have become more finely tuned, so to speak.

The description given here of the Psychic Body is a basic general one. An exercise I call "The Psychic Body Toner" is included later on to give general all-over support for this energy body. It will greatly assist with strengthening the core Psychic body anatomy. This basis becomes the "skeleton" for the more advanced Psychic Body Chakra anatomy.

The Psychic Body responds to other's positive and negative thoughts and projections.

When strong, our senses are more attuned, and we are more connected with the supportive forces of nature.

As we are learning, the body is linked in many ways and on many different levels of life and experience and when one thing is "out" or imbalanced it can have a domino effect or consequence on the whole. Dysfunction in this body can leave us feeling very vulnerable.

The Psychic Body referred to in this book is comprised of these centers of radiant energy:

> Directly above the top of the head or Crown, called The Spirit Centre
>
> At the Throat – the Air Centre
>
> At the Solar Plexus – the Fire Centre
>
> At the Urino-Genital area – the Water Centre
>
> Directly under the feet – the Earth Centre

They are linked with each other through a Central column, and can become disconnected, cloudy, gunked up, dull or even damaged in the case of abuse or psychic attack.

Using the "Psychic Body toner" as a basic exercise, focus on connecting these centers firstly, then recharge them regularly or as often as needed. Particularly when one is needing to rebuild and rebalance after negative experiences. Using the exercise as mentioned regularly initially, then as an occasional maintenance exercise, will make a huge difference to the impact from handling negative people.

The Psychic Body includes the Earth Star or *Earthing Star Chakra*, situated approximately 6" below the feet, which was not previously recognised in main systems as it sits on a different subtle body level. However, it is my opinion that including this Chakra, together with the Navel Chakra in energy work and balancing can enhance any Chakra work.

Besides these Main Chakras, there are also hundreds of minor chakras in the body, at organs, glands and joints as well as in the hands and the soles of the feet. These and other newly discovered Chakras and systems will be included in "The New Evolved Chakras". For further information, kindly refer to the articles on my website: www.myrasri.com/new-chakras-subtle-body-anatomy

More on Energy, Human Energy Fields and The Aura

In general terms, these combined bodies or Energy Fields are part of or connected and linked directly to what has commonly been called The Aura.

The human aura surrounds the entire physical body, and is generally elliptical in shape. Like an elongated balloon, the aura extends around the average human body approximately 8 – 10 feet in all directions. You are already aware of some of the major components of the aura. The healthier we are, the more vibrant and stronger our aura is.

The more energy we have, the less likely we will be to come under outside influences.

When one is in poor health, the edges of the aura can be loose, floppy, stretched, thin, vulnerable, or even scratched, torn, ripped or damaged. It can be misshapen and "blown out". This will affect the ability to regain full health, to protect our self from environmental damage or pollution, or to allow ourselves sufficient separation from the effect of problems or emotions of others.

Weak auras are more easily affected by outside influences, physically, emotionally, mentally etc. It may also mean that we are more easily manipulated, or that we may tire more easily with certain activities. We may feel depressed, or a failure or of not being in control of our life. In weakened areas of the aura, stress will penetrate or affect more quickly.

When our energy fields are healthy, charged, clear and strong, we can resist unwanted outside influences. (We are also better equipped to fight disease.)

Secrets Behind Energy Fields

To achieve this, we have to be able to sustain these energy fields ultimately and eventually *from within* our self.

Learning about what you can do for yourself becomes very important.

You can enhance your own energy fields!

You can become stronger from within! You can begin to regain the former strength of your energy fields.

The exercises and statements in this book will begin to change the way you have previously responded to others that have been bringing you down, whether intentionally or not.

To begin with, also remember the value of what is freely available already:

Sunlight, fresh air, good nutrition, healthy and loving thoughts and a little physical exercise are all extremely vitalizing to the energy fields.

For some, Meditation may also strengthen and be protective.

Others find that certain music will revitalize and refresh them, and I don't mean the emotional renderings of love songs, sad songs, heavy metal (which create disresonance and chaos in the energy fields) or really loud / high decibel music.

Experiment with some of the relaxing kind generally found in the classics, or inspiring music, as well as those tunes that put a small smile on your face.

When you are taking care of you, and nurturing you, you will become happier, stronger, healthier, and will be able to be more present for others.

Secrets Behind Energy Fields

The Science Of The Aura

The Aura and ElectroMagnetics

The aura is the energy field surrounding anything with an atomic structure. Within the atoms that comprise all matter are electrons and protons – positive (electrical) and negative (magnetic) charges. The more animate the life and matter, the more vibrant the aura or energy field surrounding it.

Auras and energy fields have been measured scientifically, as can its interactions with its external surroundings. [Early Kirlian photography developed by the Russians, had established this aura around living matter many years ago.]

It follows then that if we firstly recognize then understand the interactions that take place, we are then better able to determine how best to balance, strengthen and cleanse this energy field or aura. With a strong and vibrant aura, negative, unbalanced and draining energies are more readily deflected.

The human body also has other energy emanations as well, giving off light, sound, thermal energies, electricity, magnetic responses, heat and more.

Some of these energy fields are generated within the body, others are received from outside the body and then transformed into the body.

Like a kind of osmosis, this occurs through natural interaction between our personal energies and those energy fields around us. For example, Nature energies of fresh sea air and sunlight are easily assimilated into the body.

A WORD ON ELECTROMAGNETICS

Put briefly, the energy fields and energy centers in the body run on electro (giving off or giving out) and magnetic (receiving or pulling in) energies. These ideally work optimally when we are aligned with the <u>electromagnetics</u> of the Earth or planet. Particularly where nature is lush and abundant, we can get a positive re-alignment and be able to recharge again more easily and readily.

Planetary changes are now demanding that we take more time out in nature or to just be to recharge and reconnect back to a better sense of self again.

It is my understanding that the Earth electromagnetics have changed and increased in strength somewhat over the last 20 years alone.

This can mean that we need to increase our own electromagnetic charge to benefit and be in alignment with the Planets electromagnetic frequencies.

For some this can mean a sense of being or feeling ungrounded.

The human body has its own electromagnetic field (EMF), similar to that of the Earth.

It usually gets bathed in the Earth EMF at night time, helping reset and rejuvenate the external electrical aspects of the human body.

Referred to as the Schumann Resonances, these Earth EMF's are essential for night rest, for the sun and its solar rays are at rest from its daily impacts, and the body now has time to deal with the day's intake, impacts and events whilst processing, repairing and resting from daily activity.

Secrets Behind Energy Fields

The Schuman Resonance is identified and associated with the natural electrical impulses and frequencies of the planet in natural settings.

Some researchers believe that by producing a 7.83 Hz pulse with a field generator (using a Schumann device); we can counter the effects of these irritating man-made fields that impact on our electrical systems and our electromagnetic fields. By replicating the Earth's natural rhythm, we may be providing ourselves (at least in our immediate vicinity) with a healthier environment.

Getting away from electro pollutants as much as possible will help the body reset and feel more relaxed or 'lighter'.

If our electromagnetic system is functioning properly, we not only have better physical function in the body, we also have healthier energy fields which can often be communication systems in themselves.

You are now becoming aware that electronic and electrical devices are not the only things that can affect our own EMF. Humans themselves can have a unique frequency of their own in their EMF that can be changed according to emotion, state, agitation or a number of other things.

When we are in flow, we have less chance of affecting another negatively. When we are strong we have less chance of being affected.

Nevertheless, there can be exceptions to these generalities.

The important thing to note is that when we are around aggravation frequencies put out by others, this can impact on our own energy capabilities.

Personal Frequency, Resonance and Electromagnetics

Each of us carries our own personal personality, our individual characteristics. We are unique but we also can carry similar stories or experiences which further influence our energy vibration.

Each of us impact in an unknowing way on others. We have all met the angry person, who can make us feel somewhat tense and uncomfortable just by being near us... and we have also met the person whose being seems to simply welcome us or allow us to relax.

When we are balanced energetically, we find ourselves better able to act in accordance with who we are, and also to be around. This creates smoother and stronger electromagnetic fields (EMF's).

The first illustration will attempt to show you a sense of balanced personal wave pattern frequencies – let's call this person "A".

What may not be clearly shown is the energy output and the energy input or impact. For our purposes here, we are only looking at the general overall energy surrounding the body, including the electromagnetic attributes.

Secrets Behind Energy Fields

PERSONAL ENERGY FIELD & RESONANCE
Aura & Electromagnetics

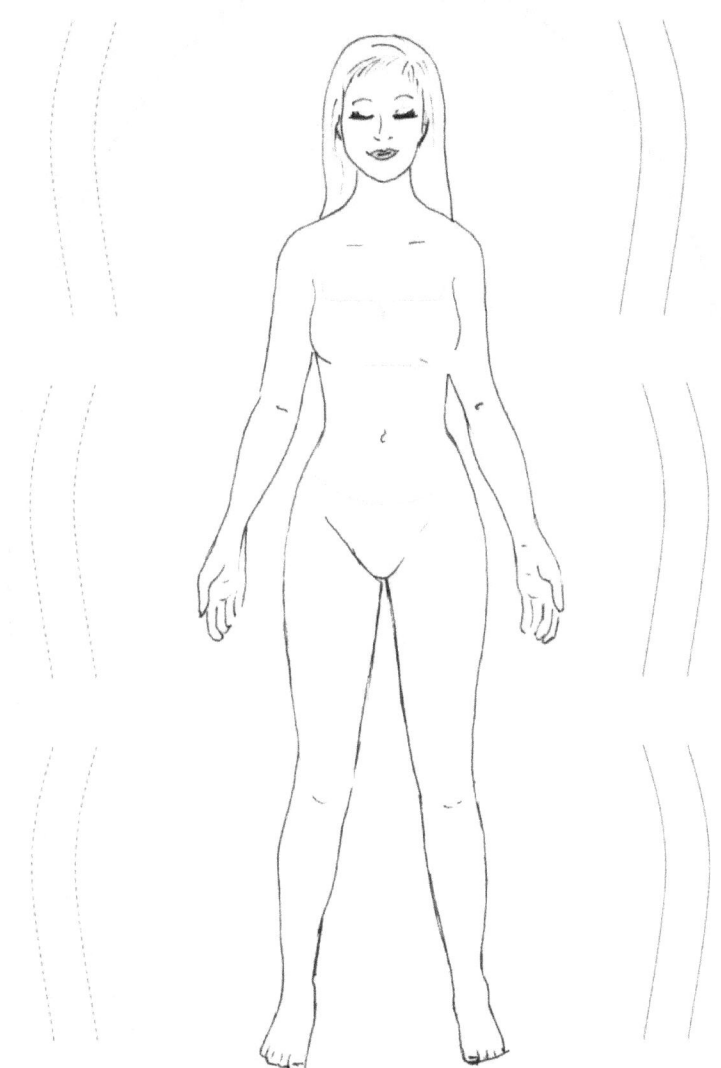

PERSONAL ENERGY FIELD & RESONANCE
MASTERY JOURNEY SERIES—NAVIGATING ENERGY

Compare this Personal Frequency image (A) with the next image of another's (B) similarly balanced and similarly vibrationally frequenced field and we may well have a form of harmony.

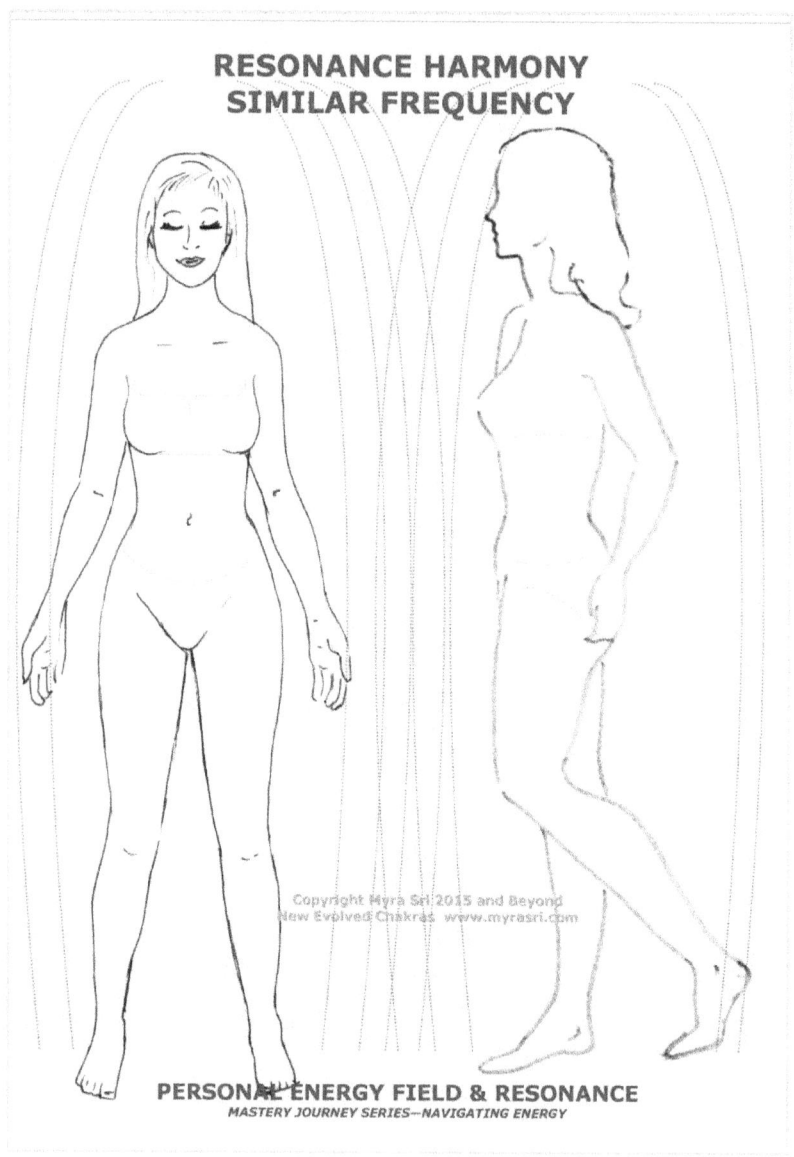

However, when another's energy field (B) carries a different range of vibrations, whether through thought, belief or emotional experience, their EMF field also carries a different frequency, and if it is different enough, it may well affect one's own field.

Secrets Behind Energy Fields

If someone else's field (B) is highly charged or more intensely powered, however temporary, it can impact and sometimes overwhelm or override another's (A) energy systems via the EMF.

This can result in change or even in control in another's energy systems.

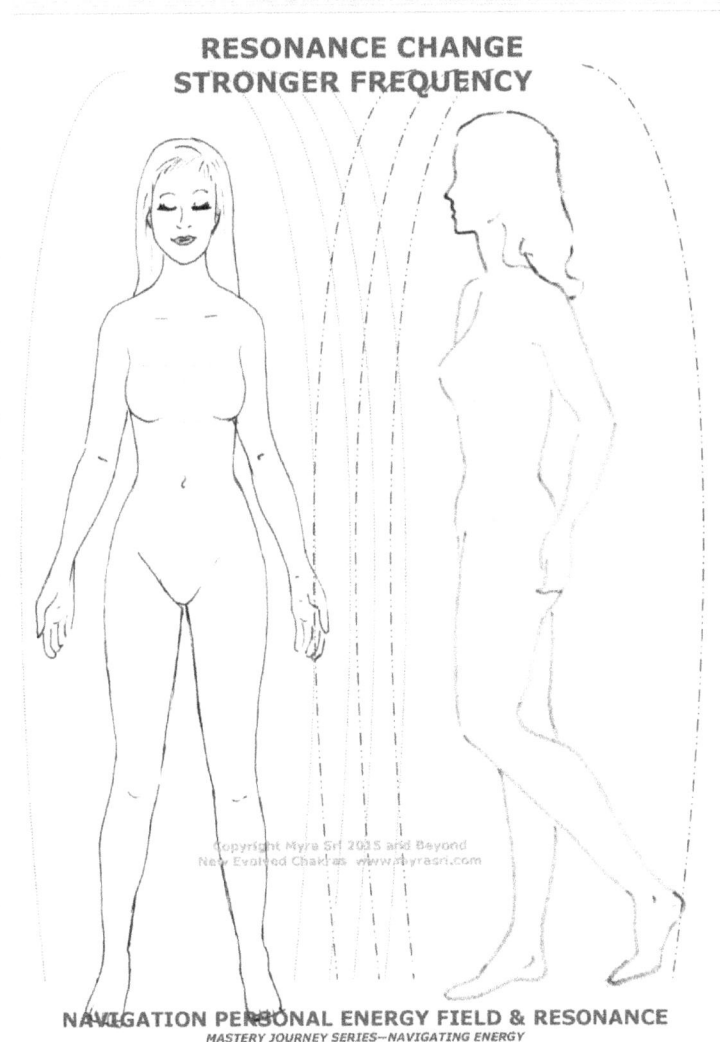

This of course can depend on the tone, strength or vibrancy of the "receiving" (A) energy field. If the tone is good, there is less likelihood of overwhelm etc, or at least, there is some warning or sensory perception of the "invasion".

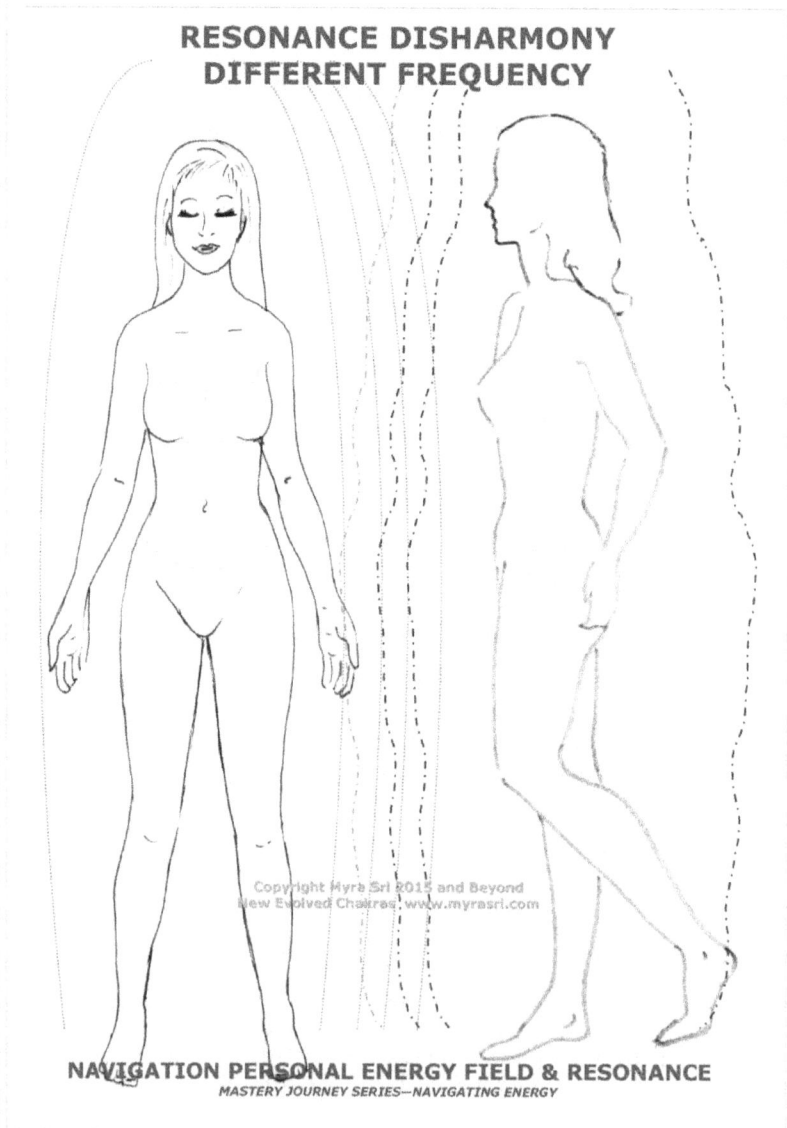

Secrets Behind Energy Fields

If the energetic impact from a stronger energy field and EMF results in positive change for the recipient A, then all is good.

In the fourth image, there may be too much difference between energy fields and so there can be a transmission of what can feel like a dis-resonant energy or simply a sense of irritation or aggravation for example, from (B) or a sense of unsettling-ness. If the difference in frequency is due to some negative emotion, memory or experience, sometimes it can actually create a similar vibration or resonance in A. This can then translate into a sense of irritation or disruption within A's energy systems of functions. On occasion, the very issues or symptoms that have been introduced by the disharmony of B can be played out in the experiences of A.

Sometimes the difference in frequency has nothing to do with what each is going through, simply that there is a possibly basic incompatibility of energy. No matter how good things are for each person individually, they may never be able to fully relax around each other simply because of the difference/s.

All of the above energy and electrical energy interchanges and interactions or impact depends on the state of the two energy fields or EMF's involved.

This is a very simplified explanation, but it can give a visual clue as to not only how energy fields are impacted, which will relate to human conditions and energy communication but also, to a degree, on how electronic devices can impact the human EMF.

Birthplace Energy Boosters

Often when we visit our birth-place, even though we may not want to live there again, something takes place energetically. Obviously if we had very traumatic memories, these need to be healed and resolved in order to appreciate the birthplace electromagnetic benefits. For many of us, we get a recharge from the land, the vibrations of the earth there, and from the possible energy leylines that were familiar to our original birth emergence and these often may help to "recharge" us again.

Having said that, having had occasion to visit my home birth country regularly, I found on my last visit that the energy was no longer supportive, but rather negatively impacting due to the many changes that had taken place.

But generally speaking, we can get an energy boost from the realignment of the energies and geographic vibrations that were present at our own birth, as these vibrations were part of our original energy blueprint or our parents.

For those of us who cannot actually visit these places, it may be helpful to do a meditation – where we can transport ourself back to those same frequencies to recharge our energy fields again.

Secrets Behind Energy Fields

GALACTIC FREQUENCIES

As we move through these current times that are so closely associated with the 2012 Mayan "change" times – a span of approximately 30 years or so either side of 2012 – and as we navigate the intensified energies reaching us from the current rare planetary alignments and from the heart of the Galactic Centre, our electromagnetic fields can become really challenged. Maintaining healthy energy fields, working with nature, taking time out for peace, fun and also for following your inner purpose and passion will all work toward strengthening your electromagnetics and your energy fields.

SEEK PEACE

Where possible, avoid areas such as the war-torn or strife stricken to keep your vibrational frequency as high as possible. This does not mean to totally cut and split from family in these areas, but for you just to be aware of what weakens or compromises your energy systems so that you have choice and awareness. When you know what may affect you, you can take extra measures to look after yourself energetically.

Secrets Behind Energy Fields

PART 2 SELF HELP YOURSELF - EXERCISES YOU CAN START NOW!

- Strengthening Exercises You Can Start NOW that will Make-All-The-Difference
- Common Reasons for Weakened Energy Systems, Energy Exercises and Secrets
- Energy Enhancing Exercises
- Proven Ways to Strengthen the Aura

Strengthening Your Energy Fields – Create Resilience

One of the generally little known (or understood) things about our energy resources and our current energy state is that it is directly related to our energy fields. For this is what reflects exactly what is *really* happening for or to us, whether in thought, feeling, action or in re-action. (Psychics and Clairvoyants can often read this activity.)

We learn many things throughout our life. Depending on what we experience, and depending on the meaning we attach to the experience, these "lessons" and experiences can become programmed into our perceptions and reactions.

Faulty, traumatized or misunderstood meanings will dictate our reactions until these are challenged and changed. If we react in a negative fearful way (possibly to something that another similar person may not find a threat) then we will weaken our energy field and compromise our ability to stay positive and strong.

Sometimes we aren't able to take time out with nature to replenish our energy naturally.

Sometimes we can't remove our self from the influences of others.

Sometimes we simply can't avoid being around certain people.

So we need to know what we can do to help our self. To know how we can feel ok again.

Common Reasons for Weakened Energy Fields

We have already looked at some hidden causes in *The Hidden Truths Behind Exhaustion* (Part 1). Now we look at things in our lives that are more easily recognizable, things that we have no control over, or that we have to endure for whatever reason.

Maybe you can go through the list below and see what has happened for you or to you in the last 12 months, or even 24 months. Unresolved or prolonged stressful issues or events can undermine our energy reserves, and will probably need your attention and some self TLC to set things to right again.

It really is worth your time and effort to check out this for yourself.

Stressful Situations or Events

Here follows a list of some issues that can upset us. They are often the result of events or situations coming to us from life circumstances or from the outside world. The following list can be used with the Self Help Tool shared in *"The Amazing Self Help Technique"*.

This list is numbered to make it easier if you want to use numbers to trace causes due to any of these issues when you use the self help test tool:

1. An operation or serious illness
2. An accident that causes us harm in some way
3. Some medications and ALL recreational drugs
4. Abuse by others, whether emotional, physical, mental, financial, psychological,

Secrets Behind Energy Fields

professional (bullying etc), sexual, or even "spiritual"

5. Shock or trauma such as divorce, loss of a family member, or of a job
6. Loss of home or high stress change in family circumstances
7. Sustained stress over a period of time over which we appear to have no control
8. Death of a spouse
9. Divorce or Marital separation
10. Jail term
11. Death of a close family member
12. Change in health of family member
13. Sex difficulties
14. Financial difficulties, in particular sustained hardship
15. Death of a close friend
16. Foreclosure of mortgage or loan
17. Sudden change in circumstances
18. Some action taken by a family member on your behalf
19. Some action taken by a family member against you
20. Some action taken by someone outside the family circle that impacts on you
21. Some decision or action taken at work that impacts on you
22. Change that impacts on your earning capacity

23. Relationship change not of your choosing

24. Other stressful situation– something else not included above

The above is to give you a basic list to start with. You may choose to expand your list as you learn to ask the appropriate questions.

You will learn to identify relevant information when you apply the secrets contained in this book. Refer to "How to Identify What Is Bothering You".

How to Manage Your Own Energy and Space to be Around Others Without Feeling Drained

This process is often referred to as "Protection" by some. Others see it as a kind of preparation for engaging or dealing with other people or situations.

In order to reinforce or strengthen a weakened energy field, and so have more energy, you need to firstly recognize that your energy fields have been weakened. Or that they are not functioning at their healthy or optimal level. Then take the right steps to increase or maximize function.

Sometimes a chronic (long term) depleted or damaged energy field may need some professional help.

Consider a counselor, a kinesiologist or a therapist in the case of a really traumatic event.

Contemplate a self-development coach or spiritual counselor or spiritual coach in the case of inner beliefs, or an experienced counselor, therapist, acupuncturist, Chinese herbs or qualified kinesiologist in the case of drug damage.

A really good basic exercise besides the Psychic Toner exercise is what I call the "Solar Light" exercise. This can really make a difference for you. Practicing this daily for a while (say a week or so) allows you to be able to get really good and quick at doing it, so that you can call on this energy in a matter of minutes, or indeed, seconds.

The key is to focus on the Solar Plexus, as this will activate and govern the energy for you, so you don't have to continually think about "holding" the light.

After you get familiar with this, you can expand the energy to include your home, your car, and your office space. Do your personal energy exercise first (see below), then just redo the exercise, expanding it to fill wherever you are (car, office etc) and then "set" the energy just the same.

Secrets Behind Energy Fields

ENERGY ENHANCING EXERCISES

Another method to amp up your energy again is to ensure that you have recalled all of your energy and attention back to yourself.

We often allow part of our energy to be diverted to others in order to help them. But over time, we don't call back this energy, and so we kind of "invest" this energy, but it leaves us getting more and more depleted. The following exercises will solve these problems.

SOLAR LIGHT - PROTECTION

Start off relaxed, standing (preferably) and BEFORE protection is needed,

Let your hands be loose by your side, and with your eyes closed,

Focus on the Solar Plexus (3rd Chakra between navel and breast/chest)

Imagine that in your Solar Plexus is a small ball of light, focus on this area right in this part of the body

Draw in through your breath white and gold light - you may imagine it being drawn in through your nose from the air around you, or you may think of it as coming in through the top of your head

Continue to draw in whilst you expand the Solar Plexus until it:

Expands to the size of a grapefruit

Then to the size of a water melon

Then see it expand further until it

Fills the torso, (take your time), then

Fills the legs, arms, neck and head (take time) – then the entire body

Maintaining this level of light in the body, now expand the energy outside the body into the aura about 18" – 3" (as far as you feel comfortable),

Maintain this level of energy around you as you set up the following three (3) important instructions:

Give it a purpose ("the purpose of this light is for.." more energy, to prevent energy drain, for protection, or as a barrier from psychic attack)

Give it a time: 1 hour, 2 hours etc

Give it the Universal Command "So Be It!" (or "It Is So" or "It Is Done!") repeated firmly 3 times.

Now you can relax, your Solar Plexus, and let your energy field take over for you. You do not have to focus on remembering to surround yourself all the time, as you have programmed your Solar Plexus to do so for you.

Note: As you practice this technique, you will find it gets easier, quicker and becomes stronger and lasts longer. Don't" try and set up the energy for too long initially, let yourself get used to setting the energy for say a couple of hours, and keep increasing it so that your practice builds up the strength of energy. Use this exercise to protect yourself, your space, room, house, even your car etc. You may find that you "overlay" (like layer-upon-layer) the protection until your confidence and ability increase to hold the energy for a much longer specified time. This is fine to do.

Secrets Behind Energy Fields

Recall and Realignment of Personal Energy

We may often unknowingly "lend" our energy out to others when they are in more need than our self, particularly if you are a generous and helpful person. It can sometimes happen with someone we care about a lot, or with whom we are intimately involved who is not well, or when they are not coping with a stressful situation. Parents may lend their energy to their children when they are sick, or to a sick or elderly parent.

There are many reasons, and there is nothing wrong with this, as long as we are consciously aware of what we are doing. A partner may also be draining us at night as we sleep. Sometimes we can become so involved with helping or assisting others that we allow our energy to still be connected to them. Or we struggle with a problem, and some part of our self is off somewhere with the problem, madly worrying, getting nowhere fast.

If we could measure our energy that is present for our own current utilization, we may be surprised to see that we are only having access to a portion of our energy (say 50 – 60%) whilst the rest is siphoned off to others or to that sick someone.

Recalling our energy back can help to prevent us from becoming sick, too. We do have the option of letting some of our energy support another, but this is best done by *knowing it* and being fully conscious of it.

We are each personally responsible for our own energy and protection.

In some special cases, we may choose to let that someone have say 5 – 10% whilst we recall the rest back to ensure that we have enough energy for our self. We can test for the percentage (%-age) of energy that is being diverted to others, and we can reclaim it fully and consciously.

A safe Level of energy to lend to others (when we can afford it and without damage to ourselves) is usually no more than 5 – 10%.

Ensure that your energy bodies are also realigned back harmoniously.

Having left a great job or a city behind, we may find we have left some invested part of ourself back there.

So it's not only with people that we leave parts of our self behind. You can test for % when you learn the amazing finger test technique I show you a little further on.

The **good news** is that we can reclaim these energies back – and this also prevents us going to others for their energy… (So preventing us from doing to others – draining – what may have been done to us.)

Secrets Behind Energy Fields

RECALL OF PERSONAL ENERGY

Take a moment to sit quietly for this exercise.

Relax and gently focus on letting your mind reveal to you where you have let your energy go. You may get internal pictures of people you have helped, or wanted something from. This may take a few minutes as your mind unravels all of the places, people and events that have claimed parts of you and your attention. Note these pictures whilst saying to yourself the following sentences. Allow those parts of you that are not yet present to gently come back to you, leaving wherever it was that they were stuck, trapped, invested or left behind. The filtering ensures that *only* your energy returns.

Speak to yourself these words…

"I now ask that all of my energy and energy selves are now reclaimed, filtered and realigned back to myself harmoniously, and my energy is now fully available to myself, with harm to no-one. So be it, so be it, so be it."

"I now ask that all of my energy bodies and energy fields are now realigned harmoniously, and my energy is now fully available to myself alone, with harm to no-one. So be it, so be it, so be it."

Give yourself a minute to allow this to happen. Some people who are sensitive, may actually "feel" or sense a kind of "shift" in themselves, they may feel "easier" or stronger as they are completing this exercise.

You can further improve the results with this by claiming the following:

"All of my energy and energy selves are now 100% reclaimed, filtered and realigned back to myself"

Retest, looking for a positive or "Yes" test response.

Recall of Selves

There is occasion where we have become involved in a project or research or have simply "split" from our bodies, allowing aspects of our self to travel far from where we are.

As we live in a multi-dimensional world, it is natural that we explore or resolve in other levels or realities.

We have many aspects to "our self". Consider that one is not just a daughter, but may also be a sister, a mother, an aunt, a member of a society, a partner etc.

The recall of all of our Selves (all of those different functions and relating aspects such as being a "sister", a "daughter" etc) back to our self, ensures our ability to be more time and space present, and strengthens our energy fields.

The statements are the similar to the above:

"I now ask that all of my energy and energy selves are now reclaimed, filtered and realigned back to myself harmoniously, and my energy is now fully available to myself, with harm to no-one. So be it, so be it, so be it."

"I now ask that all of my energy bodies and energy fields are now realigned harmoniously, and my energy is now fully available to myself alone, with harm to no-one. So be it, so be it, so be it."

Dealing With Toxic Phone Calls

These great techniques can be used when in the presence of someone who begins (or is in the habit of doing so) to whinge, whine or moan. You can also use this when in the presence of the person, or before being with a person, or simply when you are on the phone to them.

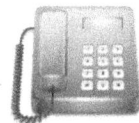

We all sometimes need to complain to others, to sound off. But when you are a sensitive person, or are already tired or stressed, you may find that you feel even worse after listening to someone else's problems.

If you know that someone with a problem is about to call you by phone, you can also prepare yourself beforehand with the Magenta Column exercise in the section on "Magenta Column or White Circle" in Part 2 in the chapter on Secret Techniques.

1. Green Ear Muffs:

Imagine that you have over both ears a pair of fluffy green ear muffs, similar to the sort of furry ear muffs worn by skiers when out in the cold. They are designed to provide a buffer from toxic words and thoughts.

These ear muffs of energy will help to filter the negative emotion attached to the words of the person speaking to you.

You will still be able to hear what they say, you will still be able to choose to be present to what they say, but you will find that the "sting" or pain will no longer be present when you listen. This will also allow you space to be able to sort out just what you can say or do that is not based on a reaction.

It can also give you more of a choice as to whether you choose to help them or not, or whether to stay involved with what they are saying, or if you want to choose to respond in a way that supports you.

Secrets Behind Energy Fields

2. Green Column

This exercise is great for a variety of problems. (I have also used it in shopping centers as an alternative to the Magenta Column, when I am feeling really tired and drained from the hustle and bustle of busy, distracted shoppers.)

Imagine and Focus on seeing directly under your feet a circle of white light, say approx 2 feet to 2 meters across. Imagine yourself standing on this. This is to give you clear space for yourself. If you feel comfortable with it, you can also later change this circle to deep red (which may make you feel more grounded or "here") or the blue of your choice, or a green.

Experiment to find which feels best for you right now.

Now imagine that the circle grows upwards and becomes a column of white light energy that comes up from the floor, and surrounds and fills you until you are standing/sitting in it – a bit like being a rose in a clear plastic tube, only this is actually the colour white, or to be more accurate, you are creating white light around you. This helps to clear energies around you.

Absorb this energy for a little while. You can do this whilst taking in a couple of deep breaths, which also gives you more oxygen.

Then you change the colour of the column to green, or even green spectrum (which is all of the colours of green that you can imagine). All of this can be done with your eyes open!

If you can, soak up the energy for a little while, and allow this energy to kind of "set". This green column is gentle, and nurturing, giving you space from the emotions of others.

A Third option

...of course, is <u>not</u> to take a toxic phone call.

But if this cannot be avoided, you now know what you can do to minimize toxic transference!

3 Proven Ways To Strengthen Your Aura, Increase Energy and Create Resilience

You should by now be experiencing a better sense of yourself if you have started performing these exercises. You already have begun to strengthen your energy fields and your aura. But here are some more really great exercises for you to do.

One that changed my life, and is really great for very sensitive people, or very intuitive people, is this one – called The Psychic Body Toner. I practiced this daily for a whole week, felt the difference immediately, and then did it for once a week for a few months and it has made a HUGE difference for me. I only use it occasionally now, when a lot of things have been happening, and when I feel a little "rattled".

This is one of the best exercises that I know to strengthen the Aura.

The following exercises are:

1. The Psychic Body Toner Exercise
2. Recognise the hidden Etheric Codes in Essential Oils
3. Use the Oil Meditation Technique

1. THE PSYCHIC BODY TONER

Each of us has our own Auric and Psychic field. In this exercise we are strengthening our connection with the natural resources around us, and this builds over time. It is Excellent for encouraging the sense of possibilities and of a feeling of "taking back power" again. It will also provide strength and tone to the energy systems that other exercises may not reach. Daily practice is recommended until you feel strong. This strengthens ones personal Psychic shield.

[This exercise is designed to strengthen your Psychic Body and to use the vitality that is around you. It has also been described by Israel Regardie, Alan Richardson, Marcia L Pickards and Ted Andrews.]

The Exercise

Centre and ground yourself whilst sitting (imagine yourself being fully in your own body, and not "spaced-out". Focusing on your breath and your heartbeat are easy ways to do this. Also feel your feet on the ground.)

Imagine a sphere of brilliant white light above the crown of your head. This sphere should be viewed as being active and abundantly alive with energy; it is your Spirit Centre and the key to your true self.

Vibrate the words "I Am" like a mantra while maintaining this visualization.

After allowing your mind to rest here for five minutes, imagine your Spirit Centre sends out a shaft of white light down through your skull and brain, continuing until it stops at your Throat and expands to form another sphere of brilliant white light. This is your Air centre, related to Saturn.

Focus on this vital sphere.

Secrets Behind Energy Fields

After allowing your mind to rest here for five minutes, imagine your Air Centre sends out a shaft of white light down through your body until it reaches your Solar Plexus and expands to form another sphere of brilliant white light. This is your Fire centre, related to the Sun. Focus on the energy in this active sphere

After allowing your mind to rest here for five minutes, imagine your Fire Centre sends out a shaft of white light down through until it arrives at your Genital region, and expands to form another sphere of brilliant white light.

This is your Water centre, related to the Moon. Focus on this sphere

After allowing your mind to rest here for five minutes, imagine your Water Centre sends out a shaft of white light down through your body until it reaches your Feet where it expands to form a final sphere of brilliant white light.

This is your Earth centre, related to powers associated with the Earth, such as food, clothing and shelter. Focus on this sphere of solidity for five minutes.

Focus your attention on your Spirit Centre and imagine it vigorously absorbing spiritual energy from the atmosphere around you.

Exhale and visualize this energy flowing down the left side of your body.

Inhale and visualize this same energy flowing under your feet and up the right side of your body to return to your Spirit Centre.

Notice that this energy is inside all of your bodies, both visible and invisible.

Keep this visualization going until the energy has completed at least six full circuits

Imagine that this energy flows from your Spirit Centre down the front of your body to your feet as you exhale, and then flows under your feet and up the back of your body to return to your Spirit Centre as you inhale.

Continue this visualization until at least six full circuits have been completed

Send your attention down to your Earth Centre.

This must be viewed as a vessel containing all power.

Imagine that your Spirit Centre is drawing this power up to it as you inhale in such a way that it fountains up out of your Spirit Centre, and then, as you exhale, it falls down all around your body until it collects again in the vessel that your Earth Centre has become.

Visualize at least six of these fountain-in circulations of power.

You are now set for the day, as this sets your own Psychic energy and assists with creating a strong Psychic shield. Really good when you think you are going to be around toxic people, or those who you feel generally overpower you.

Over time, you will find you can set this energy quicker than when you are first activating and initiating it as above.

Check here for meditations available in audio form: http://selfhlelphealing.net/self-help-guided-meditations/psychic-toner-meditation.

2. Recognise the Power of Essential Oils to Strengthen your Energy Systems

We have all heard of Aromatherapy, and we all understand what this generally means. We usually assume it is about its use in massage or by heating the oils to create an atmosphere (or "ambience") to make us feel good. When you really look into Aromatherapy, you will discover that it is also about the effect that the oils have on the human brain and the human nervous system.

Having worked with oils for many years, I have discovered that you don't necessarily need to have an oil burner for these oils to work. In fact, you no longer need to be a qualified Aroma-therapist to work successfully with them.

The Traditional Way of using essential Oils is now giving way to a more conscious or aware way of using them. Why?

Here's why!

What is NOT commonly known, or known only to a few is this...

Each essential oil gives off not just a smell, or a perfume. But much more...

Essential Oils give off Etheric Colors that do not register to the naked eye. Because of this they are also used in Vibrational Healing Systems. Each color has a light frequency vibration, and if you know anything about physics you will know that there is therefore an effect.

Each *individual* color has a *different* effect on the human energy systems. Oils also give off the *type* of vibrations that flow easily through our human energy fields.

And when these vibrations flow through physical space in a room or etheric space in human energy fields, they can create positive change.

An amazing fact is this: They can not only create more calmness, they can also be used to STRENGTHEN the energy systems!

That's right! Just by *breathing* these oils in, *in the right way*, you will IMMEDIATELY STRENGTHEN your ENERGY Systems!

Now, not every oil has exactly this effect or works this way, and you need to know the ones that do. So I have listed some the best for energy problems here for you, so that you will know which ones to use to give you the help you need.

So, number 2 of *"3 Proven Ways to Strengthen Your Aura"* is to use an oil burner as usual, but instead of simply using them for ambience in a room, now using them *consciously* to strengthen and assist one. The key to this technique is in your recognition and conscious utilization of their etheric color codes and hidden colours. Which you can consciously allow to bathe their vibrational energies throughout your energy fields, Chakras and other parts of your subtle body anatomy as well as your neurological system.

You can even use oils consciously in a bath, using the breathing technique I describe shortly. You can do this by visualization – simply relax and allow the vibrations to filter through your entire body to clear your energy systems.

You can learn more of the individual etheric colours of oils in *"Secrets Beyond Aromatherapy"*.

3. How to Use Essential Oils to Strengthen your Energy Systems

The Secret Use of Essential Oils is to breathe them in the Special Way that I explain here in the "Oil Meditation Technique".

I have seen many people who have been feeling really tired, even exhausted, who feel the lift in their energy after just a minute of sniffing the right oil for them.

And using your finger testing technique, you will now be able to immediately find the right oil for you right now!

The SECRET; How It Works:

The secret is that as the oil travels up the nasal passages, it hits olfactory senses and triggers nerve impulses that travel to the brain. This affects the nervous system which travels through the body, not only on a physical level, but on an ENERGETIC level.

Here's how:

The hidden vibration and individual sequence of the etheric color of each individual oil triggers a sequence of balancing actions. Some of the oils have amazing subtle vibrations including gold and silver colors, as well as double colors as in such ranges as orange with a violet fringe. Each oil has a unique action of its own. You don't need to know the colors, just which oil!

You can discover the right oil for you at any given time!

Just use your finger test technique that I show you in Part 3. Or simply sniff several to find the one that makes you "feel" better right now.

Oil Meditation Technique

Here are your Special Instructions for using the above oils to the best advantage.

Decide or test (using the finger testing technique) for the oil to use

Find a quiet place to relax either lying or sitting

Take off the lid and place several drops onto a folded tissue, or use the bottle as it is if you don't have a spare tissue (tissue is better)

Wave gently or hold the tissue or oil under both nostrils, ensuring that both sides of the nose take in the oil vapors or vibrations in turn. If you can, hold it so that both nostrils have access. Don't let the oil touch the skin as some may itch or burn.

Focus on breathing in the oil with each breath, but imagining that it travels up the nasal passages, and circulates round and through the brain. Then with each breath take it on a journey into the nervous system. Next let it gently flow into the organs and glands in the body. You might like to take it into the muscles and skeleton, and you might like to let it flow through every single cell in the body.

When you feel that you have absorbed it into the parts of the body where it needs it most, then through the rest of the body, now let it flow through the whole of the skin and hair, even on the face, feet and hands. Let it fill the cells in the body. Then let it fill all of the spaces between the cells.

Now take the energy that you are breathing in, and let it surround your physical body, and fill all of the invisible energy fields that you know make up the aura.

Secrets Behind Energy Fields

Keep doing the above until you think or can imagine (or maybe even feel) that your energy fields are almost "buzzing" with the energy.

When you feel or think that you have had enough, remove the oil or tissue from under the nose, and just relax, allowing the process to settle.

If you feel or think that you need another oil, you can repeat this process as above.

Generally you won't need more than two oils at a time, as they are very immediate and very powerful.

You might like to put a further drop on the tissue and if you are a woman, you can pop it down the top of your underwear, where it can give off the perfume and continue to support you (don't overdo this as some oils cause irritation on contact with the skin). If you are a guy, pop in into a breast pocket, or stick it in a trouser / jean pocket, and sniff it occasionally. You might place it in your car as you travel.

And that is the beautiful, yet so Simple and Powerful Secret of the Potency of Essential Oils.

Oils to Strengthen Energy Systems and Create Resilience

To learn more about the etheric actions of Essential Oils, there is another book available that reveals the secrets of the hidden colors held in the oils, and the secrets about their true potentials in healing. It is called *"Secrets Beyond Aromatherapy"* and is currently available from Amazon and will be available in other book stores soon.

<u>Take Note: -</u> *Here they are, but remember that <u>if you are pregnant</u>, you must please take great care with the use of oils, and check that the oil is safe for pregnancy before using it:*

Carnation   Difficult to find, stimulates and cleanses the entire Auric field, and strengthens the aura, also helps to protect from outside influences

Gardenia   Also not always common to find, but worth it - prevents energy drains, strengthens the aura, helps stabilize the aura around disruptive people and situations. Repels negativity, great when dealing with a lot of people

Sandalwood: Purifying and protective, strengthens the aura, relieves nervous tension, stress and anxiety, and helps keep one grounded

Eucalyptus: Assists breathing and relaxation, easing tensions, cleansing, good for nightmares, soothes and reduces emotional intensities, strengthens the auric field, balances psychic energies

Lemon: Cleansing, stimulates clarity of thought, used daily it helps eliminate stress from the mind and aura. Good for psychic protection

Rose: Expensive, but excellent for psychic protection, gentle. Strengthens the aura. Good for shock,

Secrets Behind Energy Fields

heartbreak, grief, depression and to soothe anger. Good all-rounder

Sage: Powerful cleanser, grounding, calming, eases stress and tension, strengthens the aura, cleanses the environment.

Some other oils that are helpful in supporting our energy fields:

Fennel Improves strength and courage, relieves nausea, settles and stabilises the energy fields after change, eases nervous tension and stress

Cedar Cleansing and protective, good for troubled dreams and children's sleep

Jasmine Relieves tension from emotional, mental and physical bodies, helps with lack of confidence or self esteem, strengthens aura

Grapefruit Refreshing and a pick me up, helps give extra energy, antidepressant, helps clear away old energy

Rosemary Protects, aids mental body, fortifying

Lavender Balances, aids sleep, protective, soothes nervous system, can be dabbed directly onto wrists in small amounts.

Secrets Behind Energy Fields

ENERGY SEPARATION ISSUES

Some Common energy interference issues follow:

- Energy Hooks
- Auric Fragments
- Soul Fragments
- Portals
- Sleep Issues
- Quick Pick-Me-Ups

Secrets Behind Energy Fields

ENERGY SEPARATION ISSUES

When one connects with others and has not disconnected correctly or appropriately, there can be a kind of hidden energy feedback or drain that can continue after the encounter. Some encounters can be less intimate or energetically connected than others. And so generally do not present a problem. However, others can be sticky types of connections, or of the needy variety, or attempts to influence or control. Or we simply find it hard to get them out of our heads or hearts.

These following three issues are the **Number One** Reason for Energetic Exhaustion and the accompanying Energy Problems. These three issues turn up again and again when I am working with others. And often they all need to be cleared together, though not always.

As you clear your energies working through these, note the shift and change in how you feel within yourself. To really register this, take a moment before doing any clearing to check how you feel in yourself first – where do I feel uncomfortable or queezy (or if indeed I feel this at all), or how clear do I feel in my head etc. This is not about what emotion we feel, but how the body itself feels – which is a good register to begin with. Then recheck after each clearing.

THREE MOST COMMON ENERGY PROBLEMS

They can affect everyone except the strongest among us, and I mean the strongest energetically. And even then, the strongest themselves can be the cause of some of these problems towards other people.

Those that are never affected may well be disconnected from others. Muscles can give some protection in physical strength matters, but not always in energetic matters.

You MUST deal with each type separately: Hooks, the Soul Fragments issues and the Auric fragments.

When you make your statement, always breathe out very clearly at the end of it, whilst imagining the hook or energy or whatever being released together with the breath. Take as many breaths as you feel till you "feel" or sense that something has shifted, changed or cleared.

Hooks

Hooks are energetic connections we make when we want to engage, hold onto, or connect with another. These are not always released when we have completed our interchange or exchange of information. Sometimes, people use Hooks to get into another's energy, or mind. They don't always know they are doing it, but it is an infringement on our personal rights.

To clear others Hooks, you can say:

"I now release any and all Hooks from others to me, and I release them, asking that they are filtered, cleansed and returned back to their source. I reclaim any and all of Hooks, and ask that these are filtered, cleansed and purified and returned back to myself for my highest evolution. So be it, so be it, so be it."

Remember to expel and release as you breathe out.

Auric Fragments

When we are intimate or very involved with others, auric boundaries disappear, and we can exchange energy without realizing it, which also includes exchanging parts of the aura. If you imagine being painted say pink, and you are rubbing next to someone painted blue or black, you will pick up some of their color, and they will pick up some on yours. To make sure that your aura is free from others "bits and bobs", you MUST return these fragments back to where they came from. We can stay connected on a soul level or spiritually, but energetically we must be responsible.

Next, for **Auric fragments**, you can say:

"I now release any and all Auric fragments from others to me, and I release them, asking that they are filtered, cleansed and returned back to their source. I reclaim all of my Auric fragments, and ask that they are filtered, cleansed and purified and returned back to myself for my highest evolution. So be it, so be it, so be it."

Remember to expel and release as you breathe out.

Soul Fragments

Soul fragments: usually when we or another reaches out on an intimate or soul level, extending a deep part of self to another. i.e. Confessions, trust, despair, desire, neediness.

And then, for **Soul fragments**, you can say:

"I now release any and all Soul fragments from others to me, and I release them, asking that they are filtered, cleansed and returned back to their source. I reclaim all of my Soul fragments, and ask that they are filtered, cleansed and purified and returned back to myself for my highest evolution. So be it, so be it, so be it."

Remember to expel and release as you breathe out.

The above can be applied to our family relationships as well as friends or strangers we may have met with. This technique will ensure that you and only you are in your own space and energy and that you are not carrying parts of others around energetically. You have enough on your plate in getting yourself sorted out. When you are stronger, then you can make different choices as to what you do about helping others.

For now, you must take care of yourself; you must be your number one priority in order to nurture your energy. No fireman worth his salt will attend a fire unless he is prepared for it, and plans on walking away from it. How else is he going to continue to be able to help others?

Prepare For Restful Sleep -

5 Proven Steps To Separating Yourself From Unsettling Energies

Review your day, briefly and then decide that you will now close all of the realities, ideas, projects and unfinished business in your mind, like you would close a book or turn off a TV or computer. Just firmly decide that you are closing them down, and that you will reopen them when you need to, tomorrow or whenever. If you have something that you can't get out of your mind, and are concerned that you might forget, then do this. Take keep a notepad by your bed, and jot down the thought. Make a list if you have to.

If you are trying to remember something, you cannot close your mind to it. Write it out and you can relax your mind easier. Close down all accesses to all portals opened up throughout the day, by worry, work, reading, watching, thinking, unwanted phone calls or any other thought or conversation activity. You can say:

"I now close down all portals opened up throughout this day; they are sealed tight so that I may sleep well. So be it, so be it, so be it."

This is part of a "Closing Down Process" which follows these steps.

Another possible alternative statement could be:

"I now close down all portals to all tasks, problems, information, people and events from this day, I separate from them, and seal them until I need to access them consciously again, and I welcome peace and gratitude for this day. So be it, so be it, so be it."

Recall all of your selves and your energy back to you again. See "How to amp up your own energy fields."

Perform the exercise "Toxicity Clearing" to remove energies that you have picked up during the day, or that you are in the process of detoxing from or clearing up.

Do the exercise on "How to identify what is bothering you" and then separate yourself from those things that have affected you. Release all fragments of others back to themselves. Very important, or you may find yourself feeling anxious from being around someone anxious when you are not normally like that.

<u>Be grateful</u> for all the good things that happened through your day. If you have difficulty with this, deliberately spend time in finding things to be grateful for. We are always better off than someone else, and so spend some time thinking about what you have to be grateful for, and focus on feeling good about this. What this does is increase the tone of your energy rather than bring it down, and helps prepare you for sleep. You are also lifting your vibrations to attract more good things into your life.

Workaholics or Worriers, A Closing Down Process in cases of Insomnia

This is a simple yet powerful process. During the day, we access lots of other realities. The term "leave work at work" may have been mastered by some people, but not everyone. Or personal problems find themselves interfering with work.

Maybe someone has an illness, or a serious problem that concerns you. Or maybe you are in the process of creating something, but can't seem to stop thinking about it when you need to be focused on something else. It's also possible that someone else has "dropped" an idea into your mind, and this has opened a possibility or other reality to your mind.

This is usually more evident at night, when the noise and action of the day begin to dissipate.

It can keep us awake at night, or create a low level nagging feeling as the mind tries to think through the problem. It also leaches energy from us if it presents a problem that we do not yet know how to solve. Use the wording or invocation of the following Portal and Reality Closing process.

Portal and Reality Access Closing Down Process

<u>Very, very Important.</u> (Also very effective after doing Psychic work or after being involved deeply in another's issues. Close off for the Client first, then for yourself. Particularly good for after mental time travel.)

"I now close down all doors, gateways, windows or portals to ALL other realities, dimensions or time-frames, with ease and safety. So Be It (x3)"

"I now Ask that All Psychic Gates, portals, doorways and accesses to All other levels and dimensions and realities are now closed with ease and safety. It is Done x 3" [It is Done repeated three times.] ['So Be It" can be exchanged for "It is Done"]

For children having nightmares or difficulty: You can get them to say something like this (adapted according to your belief systems);

"I (you can use "We" if this feels better for you both) now shut and close all the things that worry me or make me not sleep. They are turned off, closed and put away.

[You can allow the child to give you feedback as to when this is done, or guide them if they are having difficulty in closing them down – a precious time to gain insight and intimacy with your child. Then, when done continue with...]

"I now ask for an angel at the top of my bed, one at the bottom of my bed, and one on each side, please, to keep me .... (child says their name) safe through the night. Thank you, thank you, thank you."

Parent or guardian says "so Be It" x 3 to witness and support their request. You may also include a blessing prayer if you are in the habit of doing so ("God Bless so-

and-so etc...") or a listing of things to be grateful for. Just ensure that you do not engage the child's mind again and re-activate any worries if there are any family problems (illness etc). Try to keep it light for them.

Your support in this will encourage your child to develop the ability to help his or her self and to recognize when things are worrying them. This will help develop a self-help attitude built on reality and success in self protection and self awareness.

Sleep Suggestion

You can also use an Essential Oil to help you to settle down for the night.

Lavender is highly recommended, as this soothes the senses.

When I find it hard to settle down, or when my mind is still working on something, or I have gone past my usual scheduled sleep time, I put a couple of drops on a wrist and rub both of my inner wrists together. Then I put another drop or two on the wrist, smear together again and apply in this way to both sides of my temple. The Lavender oil immediately is transported into the brain via the temples, and into the circulation and the heart via the wrists, and both sites assist to transport the gentle soothing properties of Lavender into the nervous system.

But do check out the section on the Use of Essential Oils for further ideas. And practice care with oils if you are pregnant.

For the more empathic, sensitive and psychic reader, watch out for my book on the Psychic Energy Body ("The New Evolved Chakras"), which will include a whole new level of recent material and updates on the current developments in our subtle body energy systems.

An Easy Way To Clean Up Toxic Energies

The "Toxicity Clearing" Exercise is a great way to release or deal with toxic or residual (picked up) energies.

When we do a detoxing program, or change our diet to a healthier one, or even just give up something that we have used for a long time, such as nicotine, alcohol, chocolate, milk, coffee or sugar, we release toxins held in the body. Even just ceasing to use one of these things can cause the body to give off or "detox" what has been stored in the body tissues over time.

This can often have the effect of causing us to feel really crappy for a while, to maybe feel lethargic, headachy, irritable or just upset.

Not only are we detoxing from the physical body, but the energy bodies or energy field will also be detoxing and cleaning out.

The result of course, is that we feel heaps better later on, but it can take from 2 – 5 days (sometimes a little longer for things like alcohol or if we are giving up several things at once) until we do feel better. This exercise is good for helping to speed up the process of detoxing.

It is also great when we have been around a lot of people that drain, tire or exhaust us. Or for when we are focusing on a meditation program, yoga or exercise program that we have just undertaken.

Toxicity Clearing Exercise:

This used to be called the "Draining Away Meditation" as it helped in clearing accumulations within the body and energy fields. It is available on my website in the Healing Store: http://www.myrasri.com/new-healing-store.

Lying down (if possible) Centre and ground yourself by focussing on your breath, then on your heart beat and let it slow a little

With your palms up, legs slightly apart, imagine that there are valves at the very top of your head (Crown Chakra), the middle of your palms and at the soles of the feet (there are energy centres or Chakras here)

Set up a Cosmic Bucket or Cosmic Flame by imagining a bucket with divine fire or flame in a safe spot nearby

Now imagine you are opening all these 5 valves at these places (Chakras) as listed above. Mentally instruct that anything and everything that has attached itself to you, whether from external or internal sources, and that are no longer needed, wanted or are toxic in any way, are now flowing from the top of the head, down through and within the body, and out through the palms and soles of the feet.

Do this for the next three minutes. Send the energies and toxins into your cosmic bucket or flame

Now imagine the valves at your hands and feet (Chakras) are now closed

Make sure that you disintegrate the Cosmic bucket completely

Focusing on the top of your head (Crown Chakra), now imagine or try to feel that you open this up to the power of your Divine Source, or your God, or whatever you hold as the highest and best for you, to fill you up with clean,

Secrets Behind Energy Fields

clear, and relaxing energy of the very best. Do this for 3 minutes

Decide that you are keeping this energy for you, for you alone, and not for anyone else. Let this new energy be sealed into your energy fields for your future use. You will feel clean, refreshed and relaxed.

Golden Gates

Intimate relationships can be a blessing. And sometimes they can be a problem... If our energy is clean and ordered, but your partner is stressed or has been dumped on himself by others, his energy can often unknowingly affect and derail yours. It is not necessarily deliberate, though there are also occasions where we hear about abusive relationships where violence arises and physical harm is caused. Right now we are looking at energy management within a 'normal' relationship.

We are each responsible for our own energy system, and it is in our own interest, as well as our partner's, our family's or our friends, that we look after them as best we can.

Sexual activity can sometimes leave one prone to any or whatever nasty energy is hanging round our partner, so learning how to avoid taking this on can become important, particularly if we are needing restful sleep. I have taught this to many, many people, mostly women, though men have also benefited from this exercise.

This technique is specifically designed for protecting one from energetic dumping during intimacy and especially love making. It is highly recommended to create a better experience of loving and to encourage personal energy and emotional responsibility.

What we may already be aware of is that when making love, we may allow our defences to slip – to open to love (through sex) we generally often assume that we have a safe space. We have - as long as we are aware enough not to be open to negative energy.

Many people learn to close down on their feelings. Men generally have had to practice this more than women. Because of the way that men are built, that is that mostly they operate on a logical level, and they may mostly

Secrets Behind Energy Fields

mistrust their emotions (especially after they have seen females getting lost in their emotion), they may well tend to lock down sensitivity and feelings.

One of the most sensitive parts of a man is his penis. There is often a link here to his feeling nature, so sex and emotion (or feeling) can become closely connected. So, often for many men, sex can be a bit like Pandora's Box – when its open, whatever is in their comes flying out...

For some men, they have little control over it, and the various brain, hormone and nervous system reasons and reactions are too complicated to go into here.

For simplicity, let us be aware that for some men, when it comes to indulging sensually or sexually, if he has repressed lust, then this comes flying out, if a man has repressed his sensitive and caring side, this can come flying out, if a man has repressed hatred or anger, then this too can come flying out... it is like lifting a lid and being unable to control just what escapes...

So, many men (though I am aware that some women are this way too) will find that they contact their feeling side when making love. And because they (usually) feel in a safe space, they feel accepted and open to this exchange of energy.

What Happens

Be aware that when your open up to your lover's love and warm feelings, that you are also opening up to all of the associated energies. Sometimes things that have not been dealt with - baggage, if you like, from the past. The ejection and orgasm at the point of climax can carry any or all associated or repressed energies. If you have ever had 'angry sex', then you will understand what I mean. The climax can become intrinsically laden with the emotion, and the act itself, charged with unresolved feelings or issues. Rape victims can take on huge amounts of shame that the perpetrator projects into the victim, psychopathic partners can inject not only love, but also self-hatred or some other blind or unhealthy emotion. They then feel the better for this offload of energetic heavy weight, and this can bring them relief. However, the recipient can feel this heavy energy, though they may not recognize it, and feel 'dirty', 'bad', unworthy, or a similar emotion or feeling.

In some relationships, men - as I said earlier, generally it is the male but it can also be the female - dump their emotions at the same time as they orgasm. When these emotions are good, such as feeling kind, caring, loving, protective, respectful, joyful, happy or similar, then there is not a problem, and both can revel in the ecstasy that true intimate relating can bring. It is the negative emotions that are the problem. Those unresolved feelings, old feelings, harmful feelings. For the receiving partner left to deal with the 'dump' of these transferred energies and to process them, often keeping them feeling uncomfortable without knowing why, or agitated or restless in some way, or constructing lists in their head to try and bring some order back into the introduction of chaotic energies. Whilst the other partner simply rolls over with a sense of relief.

The Technique

The Golden Gates is a mental process – it is like setting up an invisible boundary. You imagine solid gates of gold that filter out anything that is harmful, that is unwanted, that is not of love or sharing or caring, and you instruct these gates to keep out all of these energies, whilst allowing only good energies to come through. Energetically you are saying 'yes' to the good of sex, and say 'no' to anything else.

Just as your partner is about to orgasm, call on these **Golden Gates**, imagining them in the genital area, and as

Secrets Behind Energy Fields

your partner orgasms or ejects, imagine them close down on any negative energy or emotions, keeping them outside of you & your energy field. Envision in your mind that you will receive lovingly only your partner's love and caring thoughts, and none of the negative emotions or energies.

If you have done the job properly, you will enjoy the love in your sex experience, and will feel relaxed and contented, which will allow you better sleep. Or rejuvenate you if sex took place during the day.

If your partner is in the habit of getting you to energetically receive or process his (or her) toxic stuff, you will notice a difference in him / her afterward, for he /she just may find that they have to deal with their 'stuff' after all. It is not your responsibility to have to deal with and process your partner's issues or emotions, and you are also denying them the opportunity for further growth. This can bring more maturity to the relationship as well. Besides which, you will get so much more out of sex yourself!

Accepting their love and sharing with them the gift of lovemaking is the best energy exchange.

Secret Techniques As Quick Pick-Me-Ups

Neck Cleaning

Magenta Column

Shopping Centre Protection

Further Support Hint

Therapists

Quick Start Recipe for Basic Energy System Support

Neck Cleaning and Neck Scarf

A yoga teacher taught me that when seeing a lot of people, you should wash your neck often, or in between seeing each of them and as often as possible. And when you do so, be aware and intentionally imagine that you are clearing the energies, problems, emotions or issues of others also.

The back of the neck has been referred to by psychics as a specific protection point, sometimes called the Psychic Gate, and this is sometimes where people may try to energetically connect if they cannot gain your energy or attention from being up front or direct with you.

Do not be frightened about this, simply be aware.

A handy protection tip is to imagine a turquoise or spectrum blue (all the colors of blue you can think of) scarf around your neck.

Or wear a scarf.

Some people use a crystal pendant to assist with this (which is wise to cleanse regularly).

Others use an essence spray or oil. Good essences to consider are:

> Shell Essence: Just Me
>
> AuraSoma Pomanders: Magenta, Royal Blue
>
> Flower Essences: Angelsword, Fringed Violet
>
> Oils as listed later in an oil base

Magenta Column and White Circle

Before you go, or if you are already in a shopping centre and (for whatever reason) begin to feel a heaviness or as though you are being drained of energy, stop for a moment; firstly find as reasonably a quiet spot as you can. If you haven't already done so before going into the shopping centre, you need to do this now.

Focus on imagining directly under your feet a circle of white, say approx 2" to 2 meter across. You imagine yourself standing on this. This is to give you clear space for yourself.

This next bit is optional, depending on if you feel dizzy or "spaced out". Imagine that this circle, is now placed in a larger square of magenta underneath your feet. Magenta is that deep purply red, like the colour of squashed boysenberries or red wine grapes.

Now imagine that the circle becomes a column of energy that comes up from the floor, and surrounds and fills you until you are standing/sitting in it – a bit like being a rose in a clear plastic tube, only this is actually the colour white, or to be more accurate, you are creating white light around you. This helps to clear the energies of others that are unsettling you.

Absorb this energy for a little while. You can do this whilst taking in a couple of deep breaths, which will also help give you more oxygen. This is not out of place, even in a shopping centre. And you can even do all of this with your eyes open!

Next, imagine that this column of white now becomes the same colour as the square of magenta, and that this magenta is now filling up the column or tube of energy right up to above the top or crown of your head.

Soak up the energy for a little while, and allow this energy to kind of "set" or settle as you have imagined it. This magenta column is quite strong energy, and will sustain you while you are in the shopping centre.

If you feel that you need to do this exercise all the time, please use another colour for more normal everyday support, as magenta is a very strong and powerful colour, and is only appropriate for "heavy duty" work. Maybe use the colour of green for your column, which helps to give you some space and detachment from the problems and emotions of others or a happy blue, which keeps you more connected with your own truth or state.

You may also change the colour of the square under your feet if you feel you need to do so. Each colour has its own property, and the only thing you need to do is make sure that the colour you choose feels right for you!

Secrets Behind Energy Fields

To Further Support your Energetic Protection

If the magenta column is not enough, and you still feel vulnerable, then do this:

Focus on your Solar Plexus area near the upper stomach – imagine that if there are any energies that have attached to you from others are not going to be cut and severed. You can place your hands over this stomach area if you like.

Now imagine that all of the energies that have attached or unsettled you are now leaving you. You may choose to see a them being sliced away from you, or being cut and disappearing.

Keep going until you feel that you are free of them.

You might want to check to see if you need to cut them from around your head (sometimes the reason for shopping centre headaches) or any other part of you such as you neck or back.

You may feel you need to use your hands, like choppers (sharp chopping knives) to actually slice through these ties, so don't be afraid to put your arms up in the air and "slice" through any places around you that you feel you need to. Keep doing this till you feel "clear" and stronger.

Finally, make sure that the color of the column you had placed yourself in earlier now fills any spaces made by this part of the exercise.

Let it help you to feel more comfortable in your own space.

When you are feeling better, be aware that this energy and light is going to stay with you until you get home.

Now go and finish the rest of your shopping.

Shopping Centre Protection:

Prevention is always easier than cure. So if possible remember to do these exercises before shopping, especially the Magenta Column exercise first. If you do forget before you go shopping, you will no doubt be reminded because of how you feel. Even so, you can still do it whilst out anyway.

Another tip on feeling crappy when shopping is to check whether you simply need a drink of water and that you are not dehydrated. Or if you are low in magnesium – our energy systems LOVE Magnesium!

A Word on Personal Protection – for Therapists

There is a clear distinction between what is called "Protection" and energetic hygiene. *Protection* is usually about preparation *before* possible toxicity, interference or contamination occurs, whilst *energetic hygiene* is the ensuring that there is no residue or leftovers *after* the encounter or event.

This is comparable to ensuring you have clean surfaces before food preparation, and also later ensuring that you clean up the cooking debris afterwards.

Or to take it into clinical situations: it is the difference between *preparing* a bacteria-free space, utensils and hospital gowns etc *before* an operation. And the clearing and cleaning up the resulting residue, toxic possibilities and dirty gowns *after* the operation. In energetic work the energetic equivalent is protecting and applying hygiene techniques to the aura and energy fields.

This is important if you happen to be a therapist, and have a stream of people coming to you, possibly venting a lot of hurt, sadness, anger or impotency in your office or space. In this instance, you must take care to clear up

Secrets Behind Energy Fields

after the session, so that not only you, the therapist, but also your next client, do not pick up any of the possible toxic energies left behind from the interactions.

If energy could be seen clearly, it would appear like "paint-bombs" of crappy dark paint splattered everywhere indiscriminately.

Sensitive people with compromised energy systems can easily assimilate these left-behind energies, and I have personally experienced this when I have attended other less mindful energy therapists. What can then happen is that the ensuing session can deal with the energies that have been picked up from what a client has left behind in a room or on the furniture and not with the current client's presenting issues.

If you seem to be working on similar issues, ensure there is no cross-contamination.

As therapists we must ensure that we deal quickly and honestly with our own issues so that none of our unresolved energies emerges and merges into the healing space.

Remember, that even if you yourself have strong energy fields, your client's may not be as resilient as yours...

For Therapists, there is another book being developed, and I would welcome your questions to include in this new book. (I may even ask you to review it for me, to ensure that it has answered your question for you and present you with a copy when it is complete at no cost.)

But for the everyday person, this more intense degree of "protection" or "hygiene" is usually not necessary.

Quick Start Recipe For Good Basic Energy System Support

THIS IS A FAST-START SUMMARY GUIDE TO GET YOU GOING:

This great exercise made a huge difference for me – it's called "The Psychic Body Toner".

I truly cannot recommend it enough... and the audio is available on www.myrasri.com.

This is great for people who are somewhat "sensitive" or even telepathic or psychic to some degree. When practiced daily for a couple of weeks, the difference in the energy fields is quite amazing.

When I discovered this, I did it for about 10 days straight, then a couple of times for a couple of fortnights, and then didn't need to do it for weeks and weeks. I only do it occasionally now, because that's all I need. It helped me get strong <u>from the inside out</u>.

This exercise, together with "The Most Common Problems" in Part 3 of this book, and the "Solar Light" exercise, you will find that a lot of problems that would normally upset you no longer bother you.

So here's the list again for you again:

    The Psychic Body Toner

    Solar Light Exercise

    The Most Common Problems (Part 3)

In Part 3, I also show you how to discover for yourself, what it is YOU need right now, and how YOU can fix it YOURSELF. This is under the heading "The Amazing Self Help Technique to Test for the Source of Problems" – which changed my life. It took me years to learn about... if I had known how to do this Self Help technique sooner

Secrets Behind Energy Fields

in my life, training and career, like I am about to show you, it would have saved me a lot of pain and bother.

But then again, I wouldn't have learned all the other great things that I share with others. Just practice it, and be amazed!

It is one of the best things I ever learned in my life and I teach it regularly to others.

Secrets Behind Energy Fields

PART 3 HOW TO KNOW YOURSELF – AND KNOW OTHERS

How to Clean Up after Others

Instructions for the easy and amazing Finger Test: your own Self Help tool for identifying issues that impact on you.

Real Energy Secrets – Your Own Personal System that will give you Your Answers!

Statements to Work With.

Disposing of Negative and Toxic Energies

Secrets Behind Energy Fields

THE FINGER TEST SELF HELP TECHNIQUE

The protocol follows, then the instructions for finger testing.

How To Clean Up After Others Have Dumped On You

STEP-BY-STEP - How To Clean Up After Others Have Dumped On You and How to Maintain Your Energy

Introducing your own Amazing Self Help Tool. This is a Proven Secret Healing Technique. Use it to Uncover the Source of the Problem

This technique is called by several names: finger-testing, muscle-testing, kinesiology testing, finger muscle test, self-test, Opponens Policis test, self-testing kinesiology, self diagnosis, energy access testing, BioEnergy testing, energy dowsing and probably there are some other names for it too.

With this technique you will learn how to discover in a matter of minutes how to identify whether the discomfort you are feeling belongs to you or to the person you are talking to or dealing with.

Based on professional training programs for advanced Kinesiologists, therapists who work professionally with body energy, meridians, and the emotion-psyche or body/mind of people, this is an advanced technique yet is so simple that if worked with correctly will give you amazing results.

Just follow the instructions here. Remember that it works best when you are honestly seeking for the truth of the matter, and not just thinking that you know the answer and wanting to be right! If you think (and subconsciously want) it to be a certain way, then it may well give you that answer, so you must pay attention to being absolutely honest with this!

The Steps

I repeat, <u>you have to be honest with yourself</u>, or you may blame the whole world for things you have set up by yourself.

1. Learn the testing process for a "Yes" and a "No" – instructions follow. When you are ready to test then ensure the following is in place before you start:

2. Make sure that you are fully present and <u>neutral</u> (you are willing to have the Truth of the matter only)

3. **Have a glass or two of water to ensure you are hydrated!**

4. Clear your mind of all other thoughts but the <u>question that you want to ask</u> (not what you fear!)

5. Recheck that you have a "Yes" response and a "No" response before continuing

6. <u>Decide</u> on the wording of the statement you are testing for (see **Statement** ideas which are given after this)

7. Ask you question whilst using the finger testing technique explained below.

8. <u>Take notice</u> of the answer given by the finger test, and write it down if you like.

9. If you need <u>further</u> information, decide on your next question/s and ask them.

10. <u>Keep to the point</u>, or you will go off asking all sorts of questions about all sorts of things not related, and confusion will reign.

Secrets Behind Energy Fields

11. Use the finger test to find out the <u>best way</u> of handling the situation.

That's it in a nutshell. Simple! So don't try to make it difficult by telling yourself that you won't be able to do it, because that is totally impossible, unless you are a total cripple.

Now all you need to do is learn the finger test technique. There is no one way that suits every single person. It took me five years to learn one particular technique. Other students just like me couldn't do it either.

Then I played around and learned of other ways and five of them worked for me immediately. Now all of them work for me and these are the finger test positions I show you here. Everyone I have taught these techniques to has found that they *can* and *do* work.

And I have personally taught over a thousand!

The Finger Test Self Help Technique

This first test to try is an easy two hand test. This original Finger Test goes like this:

Take the thumb of one hand, bring up to it from the same hand another finger, say the first or middle finger, and press together. So next we repeat with the same fingers of the other hand, and then interlink them as in the

FINGER TESTING

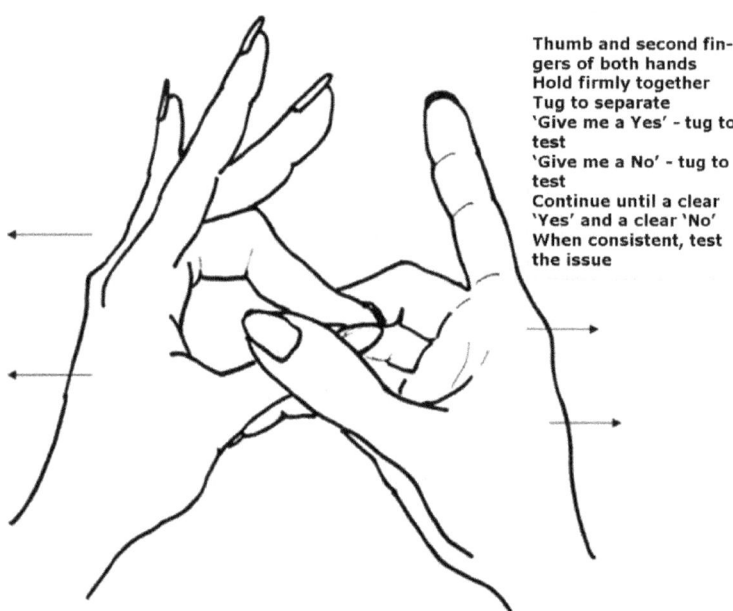

Thumb and second fingers of both hands
Hold firmly together
Tug to separate
'Give me a Yes' - tug to test
'Give me a No' - tug to test
Continue until a clear 'Yes' and a clear 'No'
When consistent, test the issue

picture above:

We apply a tugging motion and pressure to pull the hands apart, putting tension naturally on the thumb muscle and the finger it is connecting with. The pull apart needs to test in such a way that the thumb and fingers on both hands hold when you try to pull them apart.

If one finger does not hold, then try another finger, for that first finger may not be strong enough.

Secrets Behind Energy Fields

If the second finger does not hold when attempting this "test", try the index finger, which is usually stronger. Find whichever fingers can hold when tugged apart.

The stronger the hands, the fingers further away from the thumb will hold this well when tugged. The weaker the fingers or hands, it usually follows that the fingers closer to the thumb are more likely to hold strong.

We can use this "hold"ing of the fingers when pressure to pull apart is applied as the "Yes" test. However, it will only really be a "Yes" when we find that the same test is used when we say the word "No" and the fingers and thumbs fail to hold and the hands break apart from each other.

When applying the pressure (which is the actual testing process) at the same time or immediately after saying the word "Yes" gives a hold, then we can say that we have a strong test, or a "hold".

"Yes" means the hands stay connected.

"No" means that the same test with exactly the same hand positions gives way.

What we are looking for is for the same pressure between the thumb muscle (the Opponens Policis) and (any) one of the fingers so that when we say the word "No" then the finger/thumb connection slips or disengages, but when we say the word "Yes", the "hold" or grip between the muscles and the hand stay engaged and unchanged.

(What is actually happening when we get this change with the word "No", is that the muscles weaken and are no longer able to stay engaged, and the "grip" between them weakens, and so the hold is lost. This is due to nerve message integrity inbuilt with one's coherence systems as well as one's reactions to the words "Yes" and "No".

The word "Yes" is usually always accepted by the body and mind as acceptable and encouraging, whilst the word "No" can indicate a negative connotation and possibly a problem.

This system can be used in various ways to indicate when there are problems or lack of integrity via the bioelectrical systems in the body and being. Surprisingly, the body can often tell when there is a problem, even when the mind denies it.

This is sometimes termed as BioEnergy testing.)

For a lot of people, the two-hands system is easy to use for they have less "resistance" with this method, which is simply using the thumb and first or middle finger of both hands.

But if you experiment, you may find that you can also perform the same test and get the same result with every finger. That is fine, and gives you more choices. However, with men, who traditionally have stronger hand and finger muscles, they may need to use their ring finger or even their little pinkie together with the thumb to get a difference between testing for a "Yes" and a "No".

This particular finger / hand test is one of the common techniques taught for self testing in a lot of Kinesiology courses.

But wait…. If this is not working for you, there are *other* ways that are even simpler, providing you follow the method explained earlier about being absolutely honest and clear about what you are asking.

This system does not lie!

The Secret

The simple secret is in finding your own personal response.

Secrets Behind Energy Fields

What you will be doing is finding out what response you get when you ask the body (or fingers in this case) what a "Yes" response is, and that when you ask this you get a strong or locked or "grip" response every time!

Then when you know that you get this response, you can find out which finger testing position gives you both a strong "Yes" response, and also gives you a "No" response using the exact same test.

If you are having trouble, try saying the word first, then doing the testing action – sometimes there is a slight delay as the nerve messages travel to and from the brain, particularly when performing new or unusual actions.

Simple!

Now that you have played with the two hand test, there are the other ways that use only one hand for testing. And some of you might wish to do these straight away instead of the two hand test.

It is entirely up to you.

And these one hand tests are the ones I now use, because they are even easier to use (but it's good to practice on the others first to see how they work and give you confidence).

Click" and "Flick" Finger Tests

Here is revealed how to do the "Flick" and the "Click" Finger Tests. There are some illustrations included to help to guide you in this.

We start off by using the Index and thumb or Middle finger and thumb together - later you can try other finger combinations if necessary to get the clear "yes", "no" result as described shortly. For now just start off with this finger combination.

The "Flick" is achieved by imagining that you are trying to flick a crumb or button off a flat surface using your fingers. If your bio-energy response is "yes", the fingers will hold, and no "flick" will be achieved. If the response is "no", you will get a "flick".

The "Click" is similar: Take your middle finger, and your thumb, and push together.

Remember when you were a kid and tried to "click" your fingers (usually using the thumb and middle finger) to make a sound like a castanet or to signal that you had thought of something (or even as some "grownups" signal to a waiter in a way to get their attention)?

Well, that is all you are trying to do – find out which finger (when combined with the thumb) gives way when you say "No", but stays strong when you say "Yes"! (Don't worry about getting any sound with this, in fact, the quieter, the better.)

Remember the object of the exercise is to find a finger combination that *holds* firm when you say the word "Yes" and that disengages or *weakens* when you say the word "No".

So you can use a push toward the hand ("click") or a push away from the hand ("flick") - it doesn't matter which as

Secrets Behind Energy Fields

long as you can identify a different result for "yes" or "No"..

Take a deep breath, and decide that you can do this, for it is so simple once you have found the combination that works for you!

When you find it you will wonder why everyone else doesn't know about it!

Look at this picture here and try if yourself first… this is doing a finger click which you will learn to use next as the "click" finger test.

It doesn't matter if your other fingers are open or closed

Look at this picture here and try if yourself first… this is doing a finger click which you will learn to use next as the "click" finger test.

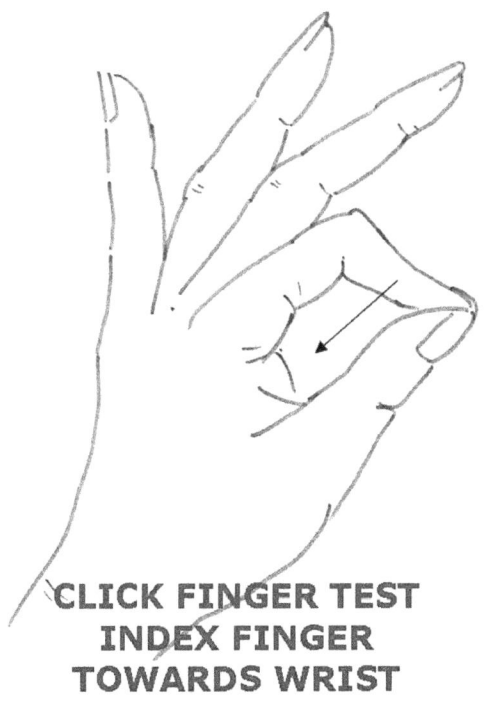

**CLICK FINGER TEST
INDEX FINGER
TOWARDS WRIST**

It doesn't matter whether the rest of your fingers are open or closed. And it doesn't matter which finger you use together with your thumb!

That's it!

ANYONE CAN DO IT!

So when it comes to using it as a finger test you will be testing how the muscle "holds" when you apply the action. You are not trying to make clicks; you are testing for muscle integrity with actual finger muscles.

And you don't need to use both hands, so you can do this one SECRETLY!

Let me remind you what is happening with the tests.

The Science of the Bio-Energy Response goes like this – when we say "Yes", it creates a positive charge in our energy systems. With most people, when they hear or say "No" it creates a negative charge in the energy system. This is not dangerous, as we are continually asking ourselves questions. It is just a bio-energetic way of measuring muscle response to certain stimulate.

Secrets Behind Energy Fields

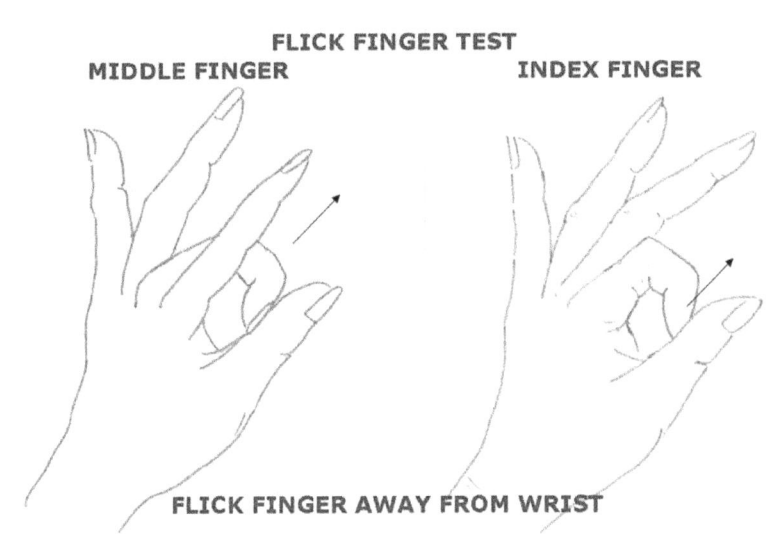

FLICK FINGER TEST
MIDDLE FINGER   INDEX FINGER
FLICK FINGER AWAY FROM WRIST

If you prefer, you may test with "Truth" or "Untruth" instead of using "Yes" or "No". It matters not to the results, as you will get the answer to what you asked either way.

Let's look at using the FLICK finger tests – check out these pictures for yourself…

This is so simple, yet many people *pay hundreds and even thousands* to learn how to get to the professional level where this technique is revealed to them! So Simple! And it WORKS!

IMPORTANT!

Once you have found the right combination for you, now you must "train" your fingers to respond to "yes" and "no" by practicing these movements. You are now creating new neural pathways that will give you accurate responses every time you need to "test". Simply give this a little practice if you don't think you have it straight off.

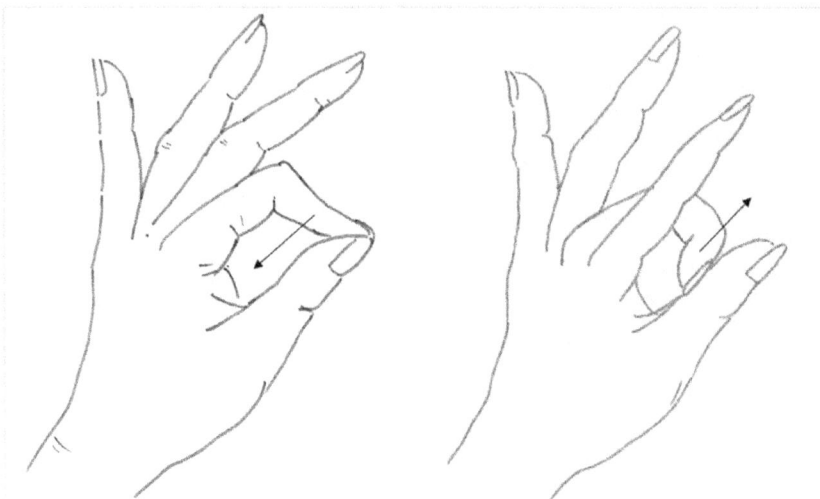

CLICK & FLICK FINGER TESTS

ALSO VERY IMPORTANT!

Before testing, always ensure that you have a drink of <u>water</u>, as dehydration will affect accuracy of testing. Always make sure that you consciously instruct yourself that now <u>you are "on"</u>. You will find in time that you can simply test to see if you are on or not. But for now, be mindful.

Secrets Behind Energy Fields

Train the Brain

If you find the finger test that works for you, but that it doesn't work every single time you test it, then ensure that you have enough water or hydration in your body. Water and hydration is super important for accurate testing.

Try again.

If it is still not consistent, then simply teach the brain-body connection by training it – a bit like learning the co-ordination required with first learning to drive – educate the brain by repeating the test like this:

1. Say "This is a Yes" out loud, then and tug and hold!
2. Repeat several times – say 6 - 12
3. Then say "This is a "No" and tug but allow the fingers to give way.
4. Repeat several times – say 6 – 12
5. Repeat steps 1 – 4 several times

Do this for several days, allowing the brain to build its own neural pathways to embed the responses of the "Yes" and the "No" into your body systems.

Then test for consistency each time. You will find that the body and brain will now recognise and provide the correct response.

A reason why this can happen for some people besides hydration issues is that they may have overcome the negative response to a "No" in the body or may have become immune to it. By doing the training as shown here you are merely educating your system to give you a different muscle test response to your "Yes" and "No".

Congratulations! This tool will serve you well!

Secrets Behind Energy Fields

How To Identify Using The Finger Test

How To Identify What Is Bothering You That You Have Picked Up From Being Around Or From Hearing Of Others Problems Or Issues (And How To Deal With Them)

You will most probably have a sense or idea that you are being affected by others for you to consider this possibility.

You may well have already registered a level of discomfort, an uneasy feeling, or a question about the person or situation.

Never, ever ignore your feelings or intuition. Let me explain here that I am not talking about emotions, but feelings. Feelings are the feedback we get from our normal senses, such as

Eyes –

What we may have seen or observed without necessarily consciously recognizing it. Are your eyes clear or itchy after seeing someone face to face?

Ears –

What we have heard, or the tone, or what has not been said that we may have observed without necessarily consciously recognizing it. Do our ears ache or feel gunky?

Feelings –

What our nerves and skin or even hairs on our skin have observed without necessarily consciously recognizing it. Do I feel clear and happy or a bit dirty?

Smell (Olfactory) and Taste (Gustatory) –

What our other senses may have observed without necessarily consciously recognizing it. Do I have a good or bitter taste or smell in my mouth or nose?

Intuition -

Put all this together, and we engage our intuition which generally works at the level of the subconscious mind. We may get these niggles or little warning signs, but out of politeness or pressure we sometimes ignore.

Our own energy systems provide further feedback, and we can get goosebumps, or feel heat or cold, or that someone is standing right next to us. Or simply a sense of something…

So having had the thought that something possibly could be going on, use your finger test technique to confirm that this is indeed so.

And to discover if it is a particular situation, place or person. Here is your formula for discovering just what is bothering you, or what you have picked up…

It is also of great importance to make sure that you are hydrated when testing, so always have a glass of water before proceeding – if you are dehydrated and needing fluids, the electrical impulses that govern the integrity of the testing will be affected, and may not provide accurate results.

Also seek to be in a neutral space in your mind – you can have ideas as to who or what is the problem, but don't try to "prove" that what you think is right, or you might interfere with the results. So adopt a "let's see" approach and you will be well on your way to gaining the benefits of this great technique.

Secrets Behind Energy Fields

ASK THE RIGHT QUESTIONS:

Having confirmed this by finger testing, ask if there is something that you already know that can help you. If the answer is "yes", then go through what you know and "test for it" until you get a "yes" answer. If the answer is a "no", ask if it is in this book. If the answer is a "yes" or "no" to any of these questions, continue looking for the answer until you find it. Don't allow yourself to get confused.

Have a drink of water before you start, and know that you do have the tools to sort this out.

Using your finger testing technique, here is a list of things you can pick up from being around others that are not helpful to you and your energy field.

Don't lay blame on them, or get angry with them. We all do this without realizing it, and you may have had the same impact on others when you have been out of sorts. This is simply about sorting through and separating what is and isn't yours.

All you need is your testing technique, the right question and this list…

So with the question in mind (framed as a statement as discussed later in 4 Proven Strategies For Identifying Your Energy Problem") such as "I have picked up from others this…" and testing as you go, go through this list to identify:

"I have picked up from others this…"

      Negative energy or emotion from another

      Problem belonging to another

      Burden belonging to another

      Responsibility belonging to another

- Shame belonging to another
- Guilt belonging to another
- Depression from another
- Anger from another
- Energy tie belonging to another
- Debris or fragmented energy belonging to another
- Energy Hook belonging to another
- Soul fragment belonging to another
- Auric fragment belonging to another

As you ask your question and test, you will get either a "Yes" or a "No. With those from the list that give you a "Yes", then you need to release them. Use this wording, or make up your own that has the same effect. Here is my suggestion, as it prevents it from returning:

"I now release any and all …. (burdens, angers, shames, energy tie/s etc) from "others"… (you can say their name if you know) and bind it to the light for transformation. So be it, so be it, so be it."

Auric and Soul Fragments are not necessary to deal with fully here. Refer to the following paragraph on "The Most Common Energy Problems" as they usually pop up the most.

Secrets Behind Energy Fields

Take The Right Action - Stay Energetically Separate:

On a spiritual level, and on a family level, we cannot be separate. We are all part of the Human race, the human family. We also live in a sea of energy, atoms, vibrations, and so cannot be totally removed from everyone else.

However, on an identity level, on a personality level, and on a physical level, we are all separate from each other, and have been since we were born, and will be until we die.

Getting the "separate" bit right whilst still able to engage with others is important for our health, energetically as well as in other ways. It is not healthy to be "joined at the hip" all the time. Or to be "tuned in" to others all the time.

We will generally (but not always in extreme cases) find that we will be energetically connected with our children, our lover or loved partner, a favored sibling or close parent.

Children are usually always energetically connected until they reach the age of adulthood, when parents should be re-negotiating a different dynamic and relationship based on mutual adult respect. Small children need this connection whilst they are building their own energy systems and connections.

Other family members that have a positive effect should not be an energetic issue, but it usually doesn't hurt to have some energetic independence.

However, in some families and in some cases there is a need for total separation, especially with ex-partners, toxic siblings or alcoholic family members etc. Otherwise you will be energetically wide open to experience second hand their traumas and dramas or pains etc.

Strategies to Clearly Identify Your Energy Problem

Using your finger testing technique, you are now going to learn to work with it in a way that will give you the right answers.

Get clear on you"re query

Questions - Make your statement clearly and TEST it

Discover - Investigate if there are further components to discover, that is if there are other things besides that are also affecting you

Fix - Work out the solution to this, from the contents in this book, or if there is some other action you have to take (for instance, not to be alone with this person again, or not to lend them something again etc)

The Steps are this:

Get Clear – Decide what it is you are wanting to know

Questions and Statements – test to find the right direction to go

Discover – by further questions

Fix – Take the right or appropriate action as indicated

1. Get Clear

The first thing is to get really, really clear on exactly what it is you are asking and what your response of "yes" or "no" indicates to you. If you don't word your question or statement clearly, you will not understand the answer you receive when you finger test. Using a statement like this, if you get a "no" response, then the statement you are testing is *not true*.

Secrets Behind Energy Fields

2. Questions and Statements

Make your statement - If you want to know if being around a certain person is affecting you in a draining way, or affecting your energy negatively or you are feeling tired, and you ask something like *"is ABC (person's name) affecting me?"* and then test and get a "yes", they may well be affecting you, but it may not necessarily be in a harmful way.

So you may get a "yes" to acknowledge that they are affecting you, but it may not help you in sorting out just why you may be feeling tired, as it could be something or someone else that is the cause of your current energy situation. So very clear wording is essential.

Another thing to watch out for is, besides ensuring that you are setting up your question for a simple "<u>yes</u>" or "<u>no</u>" answer, term your question in a way that doesn't cause you further stress. For instance, when we think about certain people, it may actually cause a stress in our energy fields (particularly if we have a difficult history with them) which may interfere with the answer. To get a really clear answer, I suggest that instead of using this question:

"Is ... (person's name) affecting me?"

"Am I allowing ... to affect me?"

You use statements like this:

"... (person's name) is affecting me negatively / harmfully"

Then test for a "<u>yes</u>" or "<u>no</u>" response.

If the statement is <u>true</u>, you will get a "<u>yes</u>" response.

If the statement is <u>not true</u>, you will get a "<u>no</u>" response.

It's as simple as that. When you become more confident with your statements and with clarifying what it is that you are wanting to know, you can progress to using questions. Until you get to that stage, stick with statements to simplify things.

Here are some statements you can use. You can also make the same statement, but turn into a negative statement such as "I am not" to gain information as I show you in some of these statements.

"I am refreshed with sleep"

"I am revitalized with rest"

"I am getting / not getting enough ... rest / vitamins/ minerals etc"

"My energy field is strong" or... *"My energy field needs strengthening"*

"My energy / energy field needs support"

"My energy / energy field doesn't need support"

"An essential oil will help support my energy / energy systems"

"An essential oil will not help support my energy / energy systems"

"The essential oil ... (lavender / sandalwood etc) is the best oil for me right now"

"The essential oil ... (lavender / sandalwood etc) is the best oil for to strengthen / refresh me right now"

"I am stressed around ... (person)"

"I am allowing myself to be stressed around ... (person)"

"I feel safe around this person"

"I am energetically weaker around ... (person)"

"Avoiding ...(task/person/situation) will/will not support my energy"

Secrets Behind Energy Fields

"My belief system around... (person) weakens my energy / energy systems"

"I am respecting myself around ... (person)"

"When I am with ... (person) I allow myself to be drained by them"

"When I am with ... (person) they drain / stress me"

"My boundaries are strong /weakened when I engage with ... (person)"

"I have/have not recalled all of my selves back to myself"

"The Magenta column helps me when I am around ... (person)"

"The green ear muffs are/are not sufficient support when speaking with... (person)"

Using statements like these help you establish where, when or how you are compromising your energy field, and alert you to looking after yourself when you engage with certain people. This is NOT about making anyone "bad", but about recognizing when you don't have enough energy to deal with certain people, or when your energy is incompatible and therefore the interaction is tiring for you. It certainly can identify when something is affecting your energy or energy systems right now, and allow you to discover what you can do to help yourself.

3. Discover

Continuing using your statements and "testing" them to uncover the truth, you now have the opportunity to get a clearer picture for your self energetically. You may discover that not only is your energy and energy systems affected by being in a certain place, but you may also discover that you are being drained or affected by something or someone else. It may not just be the one thing that has affected you. You might discover that taking a certain medication or social drug has weakened you on some level or your energy system. Or that your nutrition is being neglected. Or that you need some rest, or fresh air or sunlight.

It doesn't matter where you start when asking questions – you can't ask a "wrong" question – questions are simply a way of getting information or feedback. There is not only "the one way" to get to the truth behind your tiredness or energy lack.

4. Fix: Take Action

Having some idea as to what has been affecting you, you can now look at what will help you to strengthen your energy fields and help you to recover or to resist further energy drains.

Read again the "Using the Finger Test" section - "How to identify what is bothering you…".

Pay particular notice to the end of the list and please note that the last 2 on the list, referring to Auric fragments and Soul fragments (and the *No. 1 Most Common Problem* for energy problems). I suggest that you always start here when sorting out solutions for energy field problems.

As soon as you can, learn the best way for *you* to avoid your energy from being affected with the same situation or event or person again. Use the exercises for prevention so that you spend less time in fixing up.

Then DO IT! Take note of my suggestions in "Quick Start Recipe for Good Basic Energy System Support" in Part 2.

Or find your own weak spots and list what you discover will help you, then schedule them into your life!

Secrets Behind Energy Fields

The Secret Way To Identify What Is Bothering You

Now that you have read most of this book, you are well on your way to being able to do this anyway. You may be developing sensitivity to what is going on energetically. If not, don't worry, you are not alone, and these exercises and the information and the proven techniques in this book will stand you in good stead. You are now going to take it a little further, by learning to consciously use the finger test tool.

Using your finger testing technique, you can check when you are actually with others whether you need to give yourself any protection. You can do this even <u>before</u> you meet them, or if you think or feel that you need to check.

With your finger testing technique, (preferably) using a one hand technique you can test it quietly and SECRETLY without it being obvious. If you find that you prefer the two hand finger test technique, you can visit the nearest quiet space (say a waiting room, or a rest room) and do your questions and tests there. This will give you information that will assist you.

You can test as often as you like, if things become dramatic or chaotic.

If you suspect or feel that you are getting a bit "heady" or "fuggy" in the head being around others, try the Oil technique. Make sure that you give it a chance to work.

You can carry a tissue with a couple of drops of oil on it around with you for a bit of a reviver or support.

How To Clean up After Others Have Dumped On You – and Maintain Your Energy

The Steps

Often others are not aware of the energetic effect they may have on us. Nor are we always aware of when we have an energetic effect on others... but first things first...

When someone is going through trauma, drama or pain, their focus is often just on what is happening to them. They will perceive that they need help, and they often don't see whether this is distressing to others; and some just simply don't care even though they profess or say differently. This is not to say that they are bad people, not at all. We all experience painful things in life.

All we are drawing attention to is if or when the pain of another has affected us and what we can do about it so that we are no longer caught up in the same experience, pain or energy.

- Firstly; Recognize that someone has "dumped" on you (or not)
- If necessary, remove yourself from their space or presence
- Use the finger test technique if necessary to gain further information and the 4 Proven Strategies
- Use the Toxicity Clearing exercise to clear OR
- Use the following Disposal of Toxic or Unwanted Energies OR
- Use an Oil, with intent to clear and clean your energy fields

Disposal of Toxic or Unwanted Energies

When clearing up after being around others upsets or fears or toxic, negative or unwanted emotions, or the feelings or energies belonging to another, firstly we need to be aware of them, then secondly of how we dispose of them.

We can certainly get rid of them, but if we just pull them off us, and leave them lying anywhere, others will have to deal with the same problem later. So positive recycling of these energies will prevent these same energies in their current form from re-attaching to or invading some-one else. Be mindful to ensure the appropriate recycling of these discarded energies by using the bucket

Set up a Cosmic Bucket or Cosmic Flame by imagining a bucket with divine fire or flame in a safe spot nearby. Let this dispose of unwanted nasties and using the bucket or flame as a portal, send the changed energies to the light for re-use in a positive way. (Always dismantle your chosen imagined vessel safely and completely after use!)

When clearing residual or toxic energies, or fragmented energies, we can intentionally and consciously send them to be transmuted by the light. A sample invocation to use as a basis for this process is as *follows:*

"I now ask that this /these ...[toxic or fragmented energies etc] are now released, they are bound by the light, and sent to the ... [Divine Source/ Cosmic Vortex / Flame of God / Universe – whatever is your name for the purest divinity] for transformation and transmutation [back to positive light particles#] with harm to no one [for the highest good]. So be it, so be it, so be it."*

Remember these two points:

1. What you can imagine, you can create.

2. "Energy never dies", but it can be transformed or transmuted.

These phrases are intended as a guide to enable you to use intention to avoid further harm from nasty or unwanted energies. Just direct them and they will go.

Differing Referencing Systems:

There are various disposal methods and various destinations for shifting unwanted or unsupportive energies in order to clear, remove, transform or transmute them hygienically.

Some people find it easier to imagine the unwanted or negative toxic debris going to a Higher Power for appropriate processing. The above is just a suggestion and you may wish to use any other Title for the invocation / statement.

Others feel more comfortable sending these energies to be burnt or recycled into positive light particles via the Flame of God or the Cosmic Vortex. Whatever your intent for the clearing and whatever you feel comfortable with, choose the destination accordingly.

DISPOSAL OF NEGATIVE THOUGHTFORMS

As mentioned in the section on the Mental Body, thoughtforms can be picked up or be engaged energetically without us being aware of it/ them. But we can be free of them. The first thing of course, is awareness. So if you suspect you may have picked something up, use your finger test to ascertain that this is so. Make sure to ensure that you are "switched on" first. And to have a glass of water to ensure hydration.

The following statement can be used for getting rid of thoughtforms.

"I now ask that this /these ...[negative thoughtforms] are now released, they are bound by the light, and sent to ... [God / The Universal Source / Divine Source/ Cosmic Vortex / Flame of God / Universe – whatever is your name for the highest and best] for transformation and transmutation[back to positive light particles] with harm to no one [for the highest good]. So be it, so be it, so be it."*

*The idea behind this is to have the toxic or problem energies recycled for positive re-use or redistribution. Remember that energy does *not* simply disappear, but it *can* be transmuted. This prevents further contaminations returning back to you or from being absorbed unwittingly by someone else.

Your Secret Weapon

Your Easy Secret Weapon To Prevent Toxic People From Draining Your Energy And Making You Feel Less Than You Really Are

The Secret Weapon is simply this:

Be Aware!!!

Be aware of how you feel <u>before</u> you meet with them.

Be aware of how you feel when you are <u>actually with</u> them.

Be aware of how you feel when you <u>talk</u> to them on the phone.

Be aware of how you feel when you <u>use</u> any of the techniques described in this book.

Please take a minute to read through these again – we are so often just on "automatic", our heads filled with immediate tasks, worries or concerns, that we are not always fully aware of where we are and of what else is going on outside our own heads. But by rereading this again it will help you to get this oh-so-simple-yet-so-powerful secret weapon.

You can be aware of what is going on "right-now" without having to stop loving who you"re with, or without forgetting what you were doing. It just takes thought and a little practice.

Secrets Behind Energy Fields

PRACTICING BEING AWARE

A lot of the time, you will feel okay. Nothing much happening to cause you concern. That's ok. Learn what "normal" feels like... Now, pay attention to when you experience the following. This is the forerunner to having your energy drained, or of being dumped on and feeling sick:

You may "feel" an emotion or fear, or you may "feel" something on a physical level, such as breathing more shallow, or having to breathe more deeply. Or you may feel tension in your jaw, stomach or elsewhere. Your blood may pound in your ears, or you may feel thirsty or want to go to the toilet.

It is important that you notice what happens to you in your body, and of what you may be feeling.

If you know that you are going into a meeting, for instance, and that someone is always gunning for you, and that you actually physically register this, whether with stomach tension, neck or shoulder ache, headache, or feeling itchy etc from their presence, you can take steps to boost or amp up your energy beforehand.

You can prepare yourself!

Being prepared beforehand when you know you are going to be around certain people can really help you to manage your energy levels and energy fields. So look at the earlier sections, but also take notice of these next techniques.

Myra Sri

Secrets Behind Energy Fields

PUTTING IT TOGETHER

This section provides some ideas of statements to test for. It is by no means exhaustive, but is quite comprehensive and excellent for beginning your own journey of clarity in relationship to common energetic issues that come one's way.

This is meant as a Summary Guide and for your own further notes.

A Guide – Ideas / Invocations

Here are some questions and ideas to guide you to find out what is happening, and what you can do about it. You will have come across some of these earlier in the book.

You are also invited to note common questions and add them to the list for yourself.

Some Contaminations To Test For – "Is This True?"

It is always best to phrase your question as a statement, and test for a "Yes" or "No" to that statement.

For instance, making a statement such as *"I have picked up a burden belonging to another person"* and then test – if your finger test stays strong which indicates a "Yes" then that statement is accurate and you *have* picked up a burden from someone else.

If your self test indicates a "No"" by unlocking (or going weak), then you have *not* picked up a burden from someone else.

If you prefer to phrase it as a question such as *"Have I picked up a burden belonging to another person"* (which is a way of asking *"Is this true?"*), then you are asking instead of testing.

Can you see the importance of getting clear what you want to achieve with your test - what your indication gained through the finger muscle test means?

Always try to establish this first so you know what your muscle response means when you test.

It is always preferable to test for muscle integrity (accuracy) when you use this method to test for the integrity of a statement.   Advanced or experienced kinesiology or muscle testing can make tests in a variety of ways not covered here. Keep it simple for ease of use.

100% Testing

I usually take it a step further, but this is because I want to ensure that my clients are totally cleared from an issue, and it is a good check system to adopt. So incorporating into all of the questions that are listed in this book, you can either add this step, or simply use this testing for 1005 in all of your statement tests.

For example, looking at the statement: *"Have I picked up a burden belonging to another person"*, you can try working through these statements below:

*I am **100%** free from any burdens from others*

If this doesn't pass the test and gives you an indication of 'not true', then go through your list of possible associates or likely suspects like this:

*I am 100% free from any burdens from ... **(name)***

and go through the list of names of those you have been around or who may be involved. When you find the person, then release the burden, and release the person from your energy fields.

To check further, you can test if:

*I am 100% free from any **problems** from others*

*I am 100% free from any **pains** from others*

*I am 100% free from any **negative energies** from others*

A more comprehensive list follows:

A List Of Statements To Test

Rephrase to suit your style of statement.

"I have picked up from ... (person / another / others) ... (1 - 12)"

Or

"I am 100% free from ......"

1. Negative energy or emotion from another
2. Problem belonging to another
3. Burden belonging to another
4. Responsibility belonging to another
5. Shame belonging to another
6. Guilt belonging to another
7. Depression from another
8. Anger from another
9. Energy tie belonging to another
10. Debris or fragmented energy belonging to another
11. Soul fragment belonging to another
12. Auric fragment belonging to another

Further Statement Ideas to Test

"My energy field is strong" / "My energy field needs strengthening"

"My energy field needs support" / "My energy field doesn't need support"

"An essential oil will help support my energy field/s"

"An essential oil will not help support my energy field/s"

"The essential oil ... (lavender / sandalwood etc) is the best oil for me right now"

"The essential oil ... (lavender / sandalwood etc) is the best oil for to strengthen / refresh me right now"

"Avoiding ... (task/person/situation) will/will not support my energy field"

"I am stressed around ... (person)"

"I am energetically weaker around ... (person)"

"My belief system around... (person) weakens my energy field/s"

"I am respecting myself around ... (person)"

"When I am with ... (person) I allow myself to be drained by them"

"When I am with ... (person) they drain/stress me"

"My boundaries are strong/weakened when I engage with ... (person)"

"I have/have not recalled all of my selves back to myself"

"The Magenta column helps me when I am around ... (person)"

Secrets Behind Energy Fields

"The green ear muffs are /are not sufficient support when speaking with... (person)"

CREATE YOUR OWN FAVORITE STATEMENTS:

Create some other Statements you might like to check for yourself from time to time, and make a note of them somewhere:

1. ....

2. ....

3. ....

....

....

....

....

....

....

....

....

....

....

....

....

....

....

....

....

Secrets Behind Energy Fields

A Guide - List Of Common Statements / Invocations

"I now release any and all .... (burdens, angers, shames, energy tie/s etc) from "others"... (you can say their name if you know or have tested who they are) and bind it to the light for transformation. So be it, so be it, so be it."

"I now release any and all Hooks, Soul fragments and Auric fragments from others to me, and I release them, asking that they are filtered, cleansed and returned back to their source. I reclaim all of my own Hooks, Soul fragments and Auric fragments, and ask that they are filtered, cleansed, purified and returned back to myself for my highest evolution. So be it, so be it, so be it."

"I now close down all Doors, gateways, windows or portals to ALL other realities, dimensions or time-frames, with ease and safety. So Be It. So Be It. So Be It"

"I now Ask that All Psychic Gates, portals, doorways and accesses to All other levels and dimensions and realities are now closed with ease and safety. It is done x 3"

"I now ask that this /these ...[negative emotion, toxic or fragmented energies etc] are now released, they are bound by the light, and sent to the ... [Divine Source/ Cosmic Vortex / Flame of God / Universe – whatever is your name for the highest and best] for transformation and transmutation[back to positive light particles] with harm to no one [for the highest good]. So be it, so be it, so be it."

"I now ask that this /these ...[negative thoughtforms] are now released, they are bound by the light, and sent to the ... [Divine Source etc] for transformation and transmutation[back to positive light particles] with harm to no one [for the highest good]. So be it, so be it, so be it."

"I now ask that all of <u>my energy and energy selves</u> are now reclaimed filtered, and realigned back to myself harmoniously, and my energy is now fully available to myself, with harm to no-one. So be it, so be it, so be it."

"I now ask that all of <u>my energy bodies and energy fields</u> are now realigned harmoniously, and my energy is now fully available to myself alone, with harm to no-one. So be it, so be it, so be it."

<u>REMEMBER</u>:

In this space, you are seeking the purest highest power that you know. Come people work with their Higher Self, or Infinite Spirit. As mentioned earlier, this is a reminder that whatever your referencing system, use your preferred title for the Highest and most Positive Source or Intelligence you know. If you choose, you can simply use the term God, or Divine Source, or the All-That-Is, or Dear Lord Jesus, or Mother-Father God, whichever brings you closer to your sense of the Divine.

The important thing is to bypass normal understanding and hierarchies and go to the purest Source of True Light.

Secrets Behind Energy Fields

WHERE TO NEXT?

You are by now aware that you no longer need to be overwhelmed by the energies of others. And that you can now take steps to clear your personal energy systems from the energetic connections or residues in a mindful and easy way.

Understanding that we are all connected at certain levels is important for our spiritual growth and evolution. However, recognising that our personalities and our personal identity is ours and ours alone, and should not be mixed with others but is our responsibility to tend to and respect is important on the spiritual path. Just as we would not invite everyone into our homes and beds and kitchens, for not everyone is compatible or respectful, in the same way, we are now aware that we are not responsible for the energies and problems of others. Particularly if you are an empathic and generous person.

It is not of spiritual evolution to be continually pulled off your own spiritual purpose and destiny by the dramas of others. There may well be some learnings for us in these instances, and possibly the greater learning that we must respect our own wants and needs if we are giving out to others.

Meditation can go a long way in replenishing our energies, but is not guaranteed to clear all negative energies from our energy fields. I have seen this myself often. So it is handy to have the tools demonstrated and shared in this book.

The greater lesson begins when we are also able to acknowledge how our own energies impact on others.

Those of us with strong or searching minds may find that we create and connect hooks with others when we desire to know in order to help or to share.

A lesson for us is in this: Not to go where we have not been invited!

Basically, the wise amongst us eventually learns to bridle their own inner knowing regarding others until it is the appropriate or welcomed time to share. And to keep our energetic interferences to ourselves.

In families the desire to fix or sort for others can get us into trouble, even though often it comes from love. Allowing others to get their own lessons when *they* are ready to do so is the *real* test of love. We can be just as guilty (if I may use that word lightly and non-judgmentally here) as others in trying to make others do things *our* way, and often just so we feel comfortable about things. This is a difficult lesson to get. In the process we can impact with any negative thoughts into and onto others energy fields, and even leave hooks or fragments to tug at them to conform to how we would like things.

I have been guilty of these myself but I have learned to no longer do so. So patience and kindness is important if we want to strengthen our energy fields and only affect others energies in a positive way.

The Challenge

During my years in practice, I have seen too many energy workers and counselors leave energy hooks and fragments and even personal agendas in the energy fields of others in order to "do good" or even to "be seen to do good" or "to make a difference", and even "you need to keep coming back to see me in order to get well". These intents are not from the Light.

To be of true service is not to push what we want to do onto others, or to *make* others become our clients. And this is easily done if we have a view that they should keep coming back so that we can keep our business going…

Secrets Behind Energy Fields

This then turns from service to business and ego and our own ego fears can dictate things which can then get in the way or real clear unsullied energy help. To be of true service is to be ready and available *when* required. This takes integrity and often real work on one's self to achieve this.

The solution that helped me when I first transitioned from the corporate world and became self-employed in this way was to maintain part-time work. This way, I could shift the focus of money from off my work area and my clients and was better able to *allow* those people that needed me to come to me.

It takes a higher soul to be able to conduct and to stay in business in the healing professions as well as to "be of service" and many find that earning money in other ways can help shift the energies to allow them to be *fully* present to clients in a positive and transforming way.

Next Step

Having mastered the information in this book, and having learned how to clean up your energy fields, and those of your clients, your next real challenge is to navigate through life without leaving any of these things behind yourself.

In other words:

Not doing to others what you would not like to be done to yourself energetically.

But if and when you do, practice easily and gently recognising it and filtering back any harmful energies for transposition back to the Light again.

This is the true sign of a good healer, and a sure necessity for the sensitive or those prone to picking up on the energies of others.

A keyword is Non-Infringement.

We are *all* on a journey and we learn by doing, and by fixing our own mistakes.

Be kind to yourself.

Further Information

Disclaimer

All procedures and techniques described in this book are solely for information and personal use based on the author's research in answer to specified needs.

Practice of the techniques in this book is recommended to enable the user to gain confidence in the exercises. The information presented here is based on the author's experiences, extensive research, recognised processes, studies and expertise gleaned from a variety of reputable sources in the areas of energetic, psychic and spiritual proficiency for the purpose of energy enhancement, energy healing, self protection and personal energy support.

The author of this workbook does not intend to make any recommendations or representations that are contrary to common sense. Persons using the techniques or processes here, do so entirely at their own risk. It is recommended that one not neglect to take appropriate medical advice or recommendation in the case of repetitive physical pain or problems. Each person is responsible for his or her own decisions in the use of the material provided.

However, the processes and recommendations listed are intended to assist the reader in finding a stronger, more protected and grounded personal experience and expression as they navigate through their life and the sea of energy surrounding them.

Resources

The information in this book is the distillation of exploration, personal trial and error, research, many books, authors, energy workers and from many, many years of my own energy consulting practice and personal experience.

This book is the result of personal in depth study over the last 15 years, and has since been built on and used for the last 10 years in daily practice, both personally and with clients.

To quote all sources and trainings undertaken by me is nigh on impossible, but you can visit my website at www.myrasri.com for further reference. Additional information on the new evolved energy systems is also now being confirmed by other authors, and also by the latest in scientific Vibrational frequency reading tools and devices.

As an Author and fully qualified Kinesiologist, Spiritual Coach and Healer, Trainer and Instructor, Transformation Agent, and Vibrational Energy Healer my intention is to pass on my specialized information and knowledge to assist others in their journeying.

This book covers all the energy basics and more for those seeking to regain health and energy and to manage their energy resources better. There is more, in fact, to be written on this for those experiencing other problems, as the field of energy management is huge. Other books are planned, or you may choose to attend a workshop. Manuals to these will eventually be released.

I would like to thank my clients and all those who have supported me in this Endeavour. Thank you.

Good Health, Good Energy!

Myra Sri

Questions & Contact Information

Please feel free to write to the Author with your success stories. Your questions are welcomed and every endeavor will be made to answer each one. This book has been compiled from answering the needs of clients and through personal experience whilst training and practicing in consultancy. If there is anything more you wish to know about, then **YOU** are invited to contact me with your most burning questions as to energy, life, relationships, depression or self help, self individuation, self-identity, development or responsibility.

In return, your questions will be answered and when there are enough questions, a free copy of the resulting new book will be sent to you as a "Thank You"!

To send your question or comments, email:

admin@myrasri.com

If you would like more information about this or any other book or meditation or to be kept informed of the publication of the New Evolved Chakras book, you can email her direct, or register your email for newsletters at www.myrasri.com

Or follow Myra at her Amazon Author page:

http://www.amazon.com/author/myrasri

About the Author

Myra Sri was born in England and moved to Australia in her twenties with her then husband and two children. As a sensitive person, she maintained a spiritual leaning.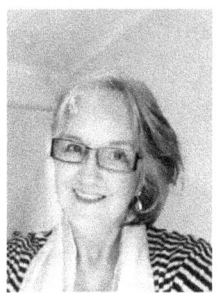

Moving out of her unsupported marriage and leaving behind her naivety in religious faith she embarked on the reconstruction of her life and the discovery of her true identity.

Continuing to work in the mainstream business, accounting and media industries, she found that connecting with other people further inspired her on her own self development journey and assisting others in their journeys led her to naturally gravitating to the healing professions.

Undertaking extensive training and study she became an energy healing practitioner and kinesiologist. Qualifying as an instructor in several modalities, she subsequently discovered where there was a lack of teaching and understanding and set upon research and discovery, resulting in her own unique advanced workshops which have been taught around Australia since the early 1990's. These continuing experiences led her to develop her own innate skills and supported her in re-membering her healing skills and psychic abilities.

Running her own private practice since the late 80's, Myra remains an avid explorer and student of evolving ways to heal and support the soul and spirit.

She wrote her first book in 2006. Regular trips to the UK concerning family issues, until both her parents died and after further teaching and training returned to Australia, whereupon Myra was inspired to document and write about her learnings, including the energy shifts with oils and crystal healing and the new Chakras.

She embarked on the Energy Healing Secrets Series in 2012 which fulfils part of her role as a Transformation Agent.

The Energy Healing Secrets Series is presented to assist in self help, self healing and spiritual mastery.

With the advent of the new era energies and her discovery of the new evolved Chakra systems, she has written and developed the *New Evolved Chakras Workshop series* which includes the new Earthing Chakras, the Psychic Body Chakras and the Signal-Survival Chakras. The discovery of these extraordinary Chakras have also been confirmed by other spiritual teachers and psychics to be instrumental in everybody's healing process and the book on these Chakras is soon to be published.

Myra provides a safe and attentive healing space for her clients and students, and works multi-dimensionally, enabling major energy and spiritual shifts. Her focus is on the Soul and spirit. Considered a resort for difficult or complicated situations, she has often been referred to as 'the Healer's Healer'. She works multi-dimensionally, enabling major energy and spiritual shifts.

Some of Myra's workshops include:

> Past Life Training – Navigating Soul Journey and Genetic Issues and Karma safely
>
> HygienEthics Series –Working With Energy, Living With Energy, Being Energy, Protection HygienEthics, HygienEthics for Therapists, Advanced HygienEthics
>
> Navigating Life in a Changing World
>
> Muscle Testing Basics
>
> Crystal Workshop
>
> New Evolved Chakra Series - New Earthing Chakras, New Psychic Body and Chakras, New Signal-Survival Chakras

SECRETS BEYOND AROMATHERAPY

The beauty and power of Essential Oils has been known to us for thousands of years, from Ancient Indian healers to current day aromatherapists.

Few were aware of etheric Colour Codes of Essential Oils.

Until now!

Essential Oils, like the Chakra systems, have evolved and Come of Age.

Their abilities have expanded and they are now poised ready to assist us all as we work with and move fully into the new energies of this new Era.

Come on a journey into the astounding colours of oils; see how they interact with human senses and subtle body anatomy. Learn their impacts and the unseen implications with the Soul and incarnational aspects. Discover which Chakras respond best, and which energy system is most enhanced by their actions. You may be pleasantly surprised!

The basic etheric body colours of the human energy systems appeared to have undergone change. Even the Main Chakras are responding differently to colour and vibration. It would seem that no longer do most of us reflect (and often poorly at that) the basic opaque paint-box-type colours previously associated with the seven basic colours of the rainbow – some of us are now able to reflect more glorious and colourful hues and iridescences from and through the auric layers and chakras when balanced correctly.

Living in cities can prevent some of these new hues and their tints from shining within and without, as the electromagnetic smog and pollution can lower the frequencies to a paler and poorer version. In these times it is becoming more important to reconnect back to nature, the land or the sea, purer energies, higher vibrations and natural remedies whenever and wherever possible to sustain us. And the essential oils is are part of this remedy.

The humble oil along with knowledge of its inherent etheric colour codes and abilities will further enhance everyone's experience of the nature and the knowing that is held within each loving oil and hidden within the etheric world itself, and will further enhance and amplify all of your current benefits when used with the increased awareness.

Recognize the New Roles that these amazing gifts from our Planet are playing right now.

Explore the Etheric Colours of over Thirty Essential Oils. Learn their Secrets.

Find new and powerful ways of working with them.

Spend time with them. Let your choice of Oil reveal to you further hidden information to assist you with your client or with your own personal transformation.

Work with Essential Oils in ways you've never done before!

Amazon Reviews:

A treasure of energetic information

Thrilled with the content of this book and I have read almost every aromatherapy book there is

I wonder why this book is not used as a textbook

SECRET TRUTHS – HEALTH & WELL-BEING

If you are doing everything "right" and yet there is something that cannot be explained that compromises your experience of life and vitality, you may well need to look deeper... look past symptoms, past the apparent, past expecting a pill to fix what you can do for yourself.

Exhaustion and tiredness can have several causes. Compromised health can often find us resorting to the local doctor or our health food store. Energetic and emotional impacts, toxicity or damage from others may need to be addressed and resolved separately (*"Secrets behind Energy Fields"*).

We are not just our body, we are not just our mind, we are not just our emotions. We are an amazing combination of all of these and more. The being is an amazing orchestration of matter and that unseen life-force; spirit. When one part is hurt, the other parts are affected.

Here in this book we look at important and often hidden contributors to compromised health and equilibrium as well as very real yet often hidden aspects of tiredness, exhaustion and depletion of energy. Many are not aware of simple things that one can fix for oneself. Nor how easy it can be to make a few mental or verbal changes for oneself that creates a positive impact on health outcomes.

If the nervous system is compromised by amalgam fillings, or lack of hydration, or unresolved issues, then results will be way short of what is possible. If the mind is blocked through lack of simple yet essential nutrients, and is not even aware of essential requirements for health, if a person cannot recognise when they have adrenal exhaustion and how their thoughts can feed into this, what chance does one have of full recovery?

Here is a mix of experiential physical advice and of energetic and spiritual tips from a long-standing expert on body-mind-spirit issues, written to help those who wish to find answers to their problems or symptoms on the *physical level* themselves.

SECRETS TO SERENE SPACE

A new look at the Art of Space Clearing. Clear Negative Energies and Use Metaphysics to Change Your Space and Life.

Become your own Guru. Learn the Art of Creating Sanctuary, within and without…

A home is a place to return to for safety, nurturing, rejuvenation and love. Does your home sanctuary nurture and support you? Does it fill you with pleasure and enjoyment?

Take a moment to look around your home… how does it reflect you? How does it feel to you? Are you able to revitalise and rejuvenate there whenever you need to? Does your home welcome you?

If the answer is "No" and you are aware that you need to do something to change your space, and possibly yourself, then you will find lots of ideas and help in this book.

If you want to go deeper than just shifting surface stuff around, if you feel that there could be some old "nasties" lying around somewhere that you would like to shift, if you feel that you would like to get clearer within yourself as well as within your living space, then this is the book for you!

Decluttering may be part of what is needed, or Feng Shui. Or it could be that there are some old or negative energies to clear. What about the sense of being "spied" on? Learn about how to remove not only "nasties" but also learn what a Portal is and how to clear these, as well as Orbs and Thoughtforms.

Discover not only how to Clear your place and enhance your home and life, but the crucial and essential step that must follow for true and lasting success in your Clearing.

Here in an easy to read book you will find how to create Sanctuary in your own personal space. These are time-proven tools, brought to you by an energy expert with many years experience. Decluttering is made easy. Imprints are explained and removal instructions are included together with further powerful techniques to incorporate into your ritual or chosen exercise to bring healing into the home.

This is a true self help book!

NEW CRYSTAL CODES

Since the huge energy shifts of recent years, frequencies have been updated in many areas. The discovery of the new Evolved Chakras has demonstrated that we are all in a process of upgrade and re-alignment. This includes not only the human subtle bodies but also the energetic frequencies of oils and crystals.

This book contains clear instructions on How to Align your Evolved Crystal to the New Incoming Energies.

The author shares her knowledge on the new Crystal Codes and Ciphers, as well as how to read where your crystals energies are at and how to align them with the new Era frequencies.

You will not find this knowledge anywhere else.

This little book also has everything you need to identify the different functions and powers of Quartz Crystals and much, much more.

You will learn about how to connect to your crystal, how to care for it, code and program it and how to use it wisely.

You will find in these pages ideas that will inspire you to love and journey with your chosen gem.

You will also learn how to identify various types of crystals, some metaphysical properties, sets of crystals and learn the difference between an Isis crystal, a Record-Keeper, a Lemurian and much more…

Make the most of your willing crystal and harness its energies for the new energy shifts right now!

This is cutting edge information and the time is ripe to re-energise your crystal.

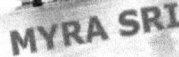